# LIVING WITH

# PAIN

## A New Approach to the Management of Chronic Pain

### By Richard L. Reilly, D.O.

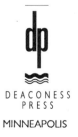

DEACONESS
PRESS

MINNEAPOLIS

Published by Deaconess Press, an imprint of Fairview Press, 2450 Riverside Avenue, Minneapolis, MN 55454.

**Library of Congress Cataloging-in-Publication Data**
Reilly, Richard L.
    Living with pain : a new approach to the management of chronic pain / by Richard L. Reilly.
        p.   cm.
    ISBN 0-925190-64-0 (pbk.)
    I. Intractable pain.    I. Title.
    RB127.R43    1993
    616'.0472—dc20               93-6820
                                       CIP

Cover design by Chuck Abrams.
Cover photograph by David Ginsberg.

Second printing: July 2001
Printed in the United States of America

For a free current catalog of Fairview Press titles, call toll-free 800-544-8207, or visit our web site at *www.fairviewpress.org.*

▲

*To my wife, Betty (typist, critic and proof-reader) and my long-suffering offspring, Richard, Joseph, Ginny and Lisa*

# Table of Contents

# Author's Introduction

▲ I'm a D.O., and that stands for Doctor of Osteopathy. People are always asking me what the difference is between a D.O. and an M.D. From a practical perspective, not much. D.O.s are exposed to a slightly different philosophy which focuses on the "whole person." As a group, we tend to be generalists, as opposed to specialists. In addition to traditional medicine, we are trained in Osteopathic manipulation. D.O.s must pass the same rigid Boards as M.D.s. The medical field is so vast and demanding that the quality of a physician depends on the individual and how well that individual keeps up with what is current in his or her corner of expertise.

I was in General Practice for twelve years. Somewhere along the line, I acquired a recovering alcoholic patient by the name of Joe Gallagher. Joe ran a down-and-out halfway house, among other things, and when he admitted someone who needed medical attention, he'd ask me to see them. I don't remember if I ever got paid, but it did give me satisfaction. I always liked being a physician. I knew next to nothing about alcoholics or alcoholism, but I began to learn. Living conditions were a bit of "God help us," but the work was good.

In the fall of 1968, two men came from Des Moines, Iowa to present a six-hour seminar on alcoholism in my community. They had started an alcoholism treatment center a few years before and were spreading the gospel, so to speak. What they had to offer sounded infinitely better than what I was used to. As part of the seminar, we were asked to attend an AA meeting. I did so along with five other physicians, the following night at the University of Arizona. After the meeting, a curious AA member inquired as to why we were there. After an explanation, he told me that if we were serious about starting a hospital program, he could raise any amount of money (and he named some impressive names from our community to help him out). Based on this lead, I approached our hospital board and was told $40,000 would be sufficient to get things moving. My newly-acquired benefactor said he'd have the money in one week. The week past, then so did Thanksgiving and Christmas. The last I heard of my magnanimous friend was that he was "bombed out of his mind" and had left the state. This was my welcome to the World of Alcoholism!

I did manage to raise most of the money on my own, hired an outstanding psychologist named Tom McCabe, Ph.D., and together with my friend Joe, started the program and called it Westcenter. 20,000 or so patients later, we are still at it. Joe died last year, and I venture to say he is now running AA meetings in heaven. He told me once that when I died, there will be an extra bail of hay for me in heaven. When asked why he said that, he replied, "all good jackasses get an extra bail." Joe made his life count.

Since Westcenter was and still is hospital-based, each patient needed an individual physician. For five years, physicians from our staff volunteered. All collected medical fees went into a fund which paid for people with no money for their own treatment. I found myself after five years with a huge medical practice, no volunteers, and a big decision to make. I had to give up Westcenter or my practice. I chose Westcenter, and I've never been sorry.

My interest in chronic pain grew out of seeing a PWCP (a Person With Chronic Pain) coming into treatment for addiction to prescription drugs and alcohol. At any given time over the past twenty-four years, I'd say that about 10% of the patient populace has been represented by that PWCP. I suspect what has been true for our experience would also ring true for other chemical dependency units throughout the United States and other countries as well. PWCPs and their unique circumstances have presented a challenge to the healthcare field that must be met.

Westcenter is located a few miles from the campus of the University of Arizona. Our counseling staff has been graced with outstanding men and women partially due to our affiliation with that institution of higher learning. Our counselors have made no effort to conceal their frustration with chronic pain sufferers. PWCPs are very hard to reach. They perceive themselves as very different from "those other people." *Their* drug habit developed through the treatment of legitimate problems. Physicians prescribed for them. They didn't take drugs for pleasure, but to rid themselves of pain. It was not their fault; it was someone else's fault. They needed their drugs. They needed tranquilizers, sleeping pills, and oftentimes alcohol to deal with life because of their pain. To most, the thought of doing without drugs seemed intolerable. How could they deal with the pain without them?

Over the past fifteen years, I started three inpatient chronic pain management units in two different hospitals based on top models on both coasts. Success has been limited. One reason is that insurance coverage is becoming more and more restricted. Another reason is that there has been no solid universal, inexpensive aftercare for those in chronic pain. When patients leave CD units, they can pick and choose an aftercare program. They have AA, CA, NA, OA, SA, or GA, and at just about any time of the day or night they choose. A PWCP just leaving a CD unit also has these groups for support, but most seem to relate poorly to group members because they are "different." Whether a PWCP has graduated from a CD unit, a center specializing in the management of chronic pain, referred from a physician's office, or simply heard through word of mouth, there's a crying need for a support system. Chronic Pain Anonymous (CPA) has always seemed a natural solution to me.

As an addictionologist for twenty-four years, I've been rubbing elbows with AA members and absorbing their unique philosophy. I was impressed in 1968 and moreso today. Witnessing many thousand of people turning their lives around through the application of AA principles and philosophy has made a believer of me! I've discussed the idea of establishing a CPA organization with hundreds of professionals, including psychiatrists. All seem to be almost as excited as I over the prospect, and I finally put my thoughts on paper and with the encouragement of my publisher and editor, produced this manuscript.

**Book I** is an overview of the Person With Chronic Pain and the chronic pain scene, surveying the problems and solutions to chronic pain. It's written for professionals and chronic pain sufferers (and their families) alike. It provides basic knowledge of chronic pain, suggests and explains some of the modalities employed in the management of chronic pain, and introduces the rationale for using the AA model for an aftercare, support system in the form of Chronic Pain Anonymous. **Book II** is more of a "Big Book" for CPA which will hopefully be used for discussion and utilization of the Twelve Steps, as they are applied to chronic pain.

I wish to point out in no uncertain terms that Chronic Pain Anonymous (CPA) does not guarantee the complete eradication of pain. Through the judicious use of exercise, meditation, group therapy, TENS Units, skeletal manipulation, massage therapy, physical therapy, hypnosis, plus withdrawal from narcotics—whatever helps—pain will be placated, but not eliminated. CPA is for those who have benign intractable chronic pain and realize they must coexist with it. CPA is for the PWCP who still has some fight left in them and wants to try something new and unique, based on solid principles. CPA is for those who want to take back responsibility and control of their lives.

In AA, the buzz word is "recovering," not "recovered." An alcoholic does not stop being an alcoholic. A PWCP, by definition, does not stop having pain. An alcoholic is one drink away from his or her next drunk, and a PWCP is often one pill, one tantrum, one lapse of discipline away from blowing it, too. Strength comes from AA; strength for the PWCP will come from CPA. It takes much hard work to turn your life around, but it beats any alternative.

I'd like to acknowledge the fact that I had a great editor for the material presented. His name is Jay Johnson. When I see and have seen so many PWCPs who need help, I have a tendency to get carried away and lose objectivity. Jay kept me focused and offered valuable assistance, particularly in a literary sense.

If one person's life is positively influenced by this work, it will have been worth the effort putting this book together. Remember my friend, Joe Gallagher? I made that same statement to Joe when we first started Westcenter. Joe laughed and said, "That's dumb. We're going to help *thousands* of people!" He was right. Joe didn't graduate from high school, but he was much smarter and had more wisdom than most people. Of course, Joe had the advantage of forty years of practicing the principles and philosophy of AA. That was his edge. I hope your halo fits, Joe . . . and make sure that bale of hay is fresh.  ▲

Richard Reilly

▲ We would like to thank Alcoholics Anonymous (AA) for allowing us to adapt their Twelve Steps and Twelve Traditions for chronic benign intractable pain and related pain disorders.

## The 12 Steps of A.A.

1. We admitted we were powerless over alcohol—that our lives had become unmanageable.

2. Came to believe that a Power greater than ourselves could restore us to sanity.

3. Made a decision to turn our will and our lives over to the care of God, AS WE UNDERSTOOD HIM.

4. Made a searching and fearless moral inventory of ourselves.

5. Admitted to God, to ourselves and to another human being the exact nature of our wrongs.

6. Were entirely ready to have God remove all these defects of character.

7. Humbly asked Him to remove our shortcomings.

8. Made a list of all persons we had harmed, and became willing to make amends to them all.

9. Made direct amends to such people wherever possible, except when to do so would injure them or others.

10. Continued to take personal inventory and when we were wrong promptly admitted it.

11. Sought through prayer and meditation to improve our conscious contact with God AS WE UNDERSTOOD HIM, praying only for knowledge of His will for us and the power to carry that out.

12. Having had a spiritual awakening as the result of these steps, we tried to carry this message to alcoholics, and to practice these principles in all our affairs.

# Book I

## Problems and Solutions

# Pain—Just What Is It?

▲   It's a simple question, but with a difficult answer. We're able to describe pain graphically enough. Our vocabularies fill that bill admirably. Pain can be fleeting, constant, grinding, stabbing, biting, lancinating, excruciating, throbbing, crushing, burning, unremitting, boring, pounding, tormenting, unbearable, agonizing, and so on. Defining it, however, is more troublesome.

*Webster's New World Dictionary* defines pain as "a sensation of hurting or strong discomfort in some part of the body caused by injury or disease or dysfunctional disorder and transmitted through the nervous system." Actually this is but one of hundreds of pain definitions. Another reads, "Pain is a sensory experience evoked by stimuli that injure or threaten to destroy tissue defined introspectively by every man that hurts." Perhaps the simplest definition of pain is "anything that hurts."

Pain is not only hard to define, it's also hard to assess. It's not impossible to quantify pain accurately, but because everyone experiences pain differently, it's most difficult. There are too many factors that influence it. Pain is a complex, personal experience which may or may not correlate to the extent of a person's bodily injury. Pain is altered by psychosocial, ethnic, biological, physiological, and chemical factors. Frankly most people could care less how pain is defined, whether it's subjective, objective, a sensation, or a perception—what they *are* interested in is getting rid of it.

## Acute vs. Chronic

In discussing pain, it's most important to differentiate between the terms acute and chronic. *Acute* pain is self-limited. In terms of time, acute pain lasts about one month, no more. After the month, the appropriate term is *sub-acute* pain. After six months, the pain is referred to as *chronic.* With acute and sub-acute pain, there is hope for relief, a light at the end of the tunnel; with chronic pain (or *chronic benign intractable pain*) the light is attached to the proverbial oncoming train. Once you cross into the "no man's land" of chronic pain, a whole new, frustrating world opens from which there is practically no hope of recovery, only a state of "recovering." If you suffer from chronic pain, you'll either have to learn to live and cope with the pain or it will totally destroy you.

The treatments for acute and chronic pain are entirely different. Acute pain is managed by using narcotics and other analgesics, nerve blocks, electrical stimulation, or surgical procedures, all with the definitive goal of discovering and eliminating the nociceptive (painful) input. Drugs and procedures "fix" it. A boil, for instance, may be very painful; drainage and antibiotics "fix" it. An appendectomy surgically "fixes" an appendicitis. When a broken bone heals the pain usually leaves. When an ulcer heals, the pain goes away. Chronic pain, in contrast, doesn't go away.

Acute pain is unwelcome, sometimes incapacitating and often financially costly, but it seldom fouls up your life. Chronic pain does. It is rare to see a patient with acute pain become *addicted* to narcotics, tranquilizers, sleeping pills, or other medications; addiction is extremely common for patients with chronic pain. Probably 50 to 70% of People With Chronic Pain (or PWCPs) become cross-addicted to multiple drugs, including alcohol. Situational depression is common to both acute and chronic pain sufferers, but PWCPs tend to be much worse. People with chronic benign intractable pain have much to be depressed about.

The behavioral management of chronic pain is entirely different from acute and sub-acute pain. Behavioral modification is the cornerstone in addressing chronic pain, and it has little to do with treating other types of pain. The primary goal in the treatment of chronic pain is to achieve reasonable function for the patient while allowing for some semblance of comfort. At the same time, the goal is to hopefully decrease the level of pain. A secondary goal is to lessen the PWCP's dependency on the healthcare system. This information is obviously dismal and unwelcome news for the patient with chronic pain, a person who naturally expects *complete* pain relief.

Here is perhaps the most important difference between the treatment of acute and chronic pain: the amelioration of acute pain is usually delivered by someone or something other than the patient. In chronic cases, however, the alleviation of pain is largely due to individuals accepting responsibility for their own pain and managing the pain for themselves. Acute and sub-acute pain relief is delivered from without; relief from chronic pain primarily comes from within.

## Cancer

Patients with advanced cases of cancer often experience horrible chronic pain, but we differentiate the pain due to cancer from chronic benign intractable pain. The pain from terminal cancer is entirely different from chronic benign intractable pain. The goals and management procedures are different in both cases.

The goal in the management of pain connected with terminal cancer is *palliative* or masking. The primary objective is to allow a patient to die in reasonable comfort with a maximum amount of dignity. Everything is orientated to that end—the optimal use of narcotics and other mind-altering agents, the employment of any reasonable surgical procedures, the use of electrical appliances, and whatever else it takes is the order of the day. Behavior modification is placed on the back burner. Addiction is rarely considered.

## What Causes Acute Pain?

Anything in your body that results in cellular breakdown with the resultant liberation of noxious biochemical substances will start the pain process. Surgical procedures, blunt trauma, disease, inflammation, and any number of injuries can cause the release of noxious biochemicals from body tissues. Biochemicals such as substance "P," prostaglandins, bradykins, leukotrienes, potassium and many more, activate special receptors called *nociceptors.* Excitation of nociceptors cause an impulse to be transmitted to your central nervous system. Specialized nociceptors are located all over the body, in your skin, muscles, tendons, soft tissue, intestines, bones, and most of the internal organs. You have these nerve receptors in your body for a reason. They are your connection with the outside world. They are the initial collectors of information that is fired off to the brain. These specialized pain receptors help save lives. They help save tissue, and warn us when something is wrong out there in the periphery. They tell you that your skin is being burned, your leg is broken, your joints are not right, a particle is in the eye, you have a stomach ulcer, it's cold outside, something is pressing on a nerve, there's a lack of blood supply, and so on. Without the benefit of these special nerve receptors, it would be extremely unlikely that we would have survived long as a species.

The "pain impulse" chemically starts in the periphery tissues and is carried by specialized nerves to the spinal canal. From there, the pain "message" is transferred to the brain. Some nerve fibers transmit their signals very fast, others slowly; some are "insulated," while some are not. The sensory nerve fibers converge in the tissues in the periphery of the body as they progress to their termination in the spinal cord. As the nerves converge, they join other nerves and become larger in size, much like streams flow into each other and become rivers.

The physical "nerve," as you most often think of it, is actually the extension of a nerve cell or neuron. It is an antennae of the neuron. The neuron may send these extensions or antennae in any number of directions. Some of these extensions are so fine they can be identified only by extremely powerful microscopes; others are easily seen by the naked eye and are several feet in length. As the thickened nerve approaches the spinal cord, connections are made in the dorsal root ganglia which is located in the back portion of the skeletal spine. This is the home for small neurons which give rise to unmyelinated (uncoated or uninsulated) and thinly myelinated axons (extensions which carry pain impulses). The neurons in the dorsal root ganglion send the pain message through individual openings provided by the vertebra, and they terminate in the back of the spinal cord in a place called the dorsal horn.

The dorsal horn is composed of layers. The larger "A" fibers connect in the deeper layers or laminae. The small, thinner fibers, which account for most pain-carrying fibers, terminate in more superficial layers. Apparently many interconnections take place in the dorsal horn which may account for an *inhibition* of the transfer of pain messages up the spine. The interconnections in this area represent a rich source of research by neurophysiologists. Many physiologists recognize this special area as a place where pain might definitely be influenced by specific electrical and chemical activity. How the inhibition of pain takes place in the dorsal horn area is the source of furious study which could eventually result in significant strides in the field of pain management.

Before the pain message is sent up the spine, about 70 to 80% of the fibers cross over to the other side of the spinal cord. These fibers are usually located in either the spinothalamic or the paleospinothalamic tract. The spinothalamic tract is relatively superficial; the paleospinothalamic tract is deep in the cord. As evidenced by the names of the tracts, they run up the spine and about half of them terminate in the brain's thalamus region. Branches of the rest of the fibers terminate along the way up the spine. The thalamus sorts out the messages and sends the impulse to the appropriate terminal in the brain. The brain does the interpretation, with the thalamus acting as a sort of computer relay station.

The nerve impulses are not transferred from nerve

to nerve by accident. The stimulation of the receptor cells out in the periphery and the eventual transfer of the pain message to the end point in the brain is not accomplished by one long nerve. The impulse is transferred many, many times from one nerve to another nerve along the way. The place where the transfer occurs is called a *synapse* and it's the site of a specific chemical process. The impulse hits the end of the nerve and it releases selective substances called neurotransmitters. These neurotransmitters react with specific receptors on an adjacent nerve which produces a certain physiological response. There are many neurotransmitters, and anything that alters the quantity of neurotransmitters through processes like destruction, development, re-uptake, or production will have a profound effect on the efficiency of the nervous system. For instance, the action of Prozac, a widely-prescribed drug for depression, is presumed to be linked with its inhibition of the system's uptake of the neurotransmitter serotonin.

## Blocking Pain

Several interesting studies have evolved recently, centering around the neurotransmitters and pain. Substance "P," for instance, is a major chemical transmitter for pain. Endorphins, which are produced by the body, can take the place of substance "P" in the synapse where the nerve impulse is passed along. Neurotransmitters like endorphins act like keys that fit into locks. When endorphins are substituted for substance "P," it apparently halts or modifies the pain impulse. Anything that enhances the production of endorphins, like exercise, biofeedback, or meditation, will indeed modify pain. Endorphins, pound for pound, are ten times stronger than morphine. If endorphins numerically outnumber substance "P" at the nerve receptor sites, then pain stops. This process takes place without the use of drugs. The body, and more specifically the mind, is therefore capable of stopping pain.

The "Gate" theory is another interesting story. The theory was promoted by Ronald Melzak, M.D. and Patrick Wall, M.D. in 1965. They postulated that inhibitory fibers, or fibers that could halt pain messages, branch out from the large "A" fibers in the substantia gelatinosa of the dorsal horn of the gray matter (the gray matter composes the inner core of nerve tissue in the central nervous system, divided into ten layers or lamina). These are the same fibers that come from the periphery and eventually form the dorsal columns of the spinal cord. Stimulation of the large fibers closes the "gate" of pain messages through inhibition. This blocks transmission beyond the point of painful "noxious input."

The Gate theory revolutionized the pain treatment business. The next big breakthrough came in 1975 when Hughes and Kostelitz discovered enkephalins and endorphins. Since then, over sixty neurotransmitters have been isolated. Understanding each physical component can help break the transmission of pain messages. It was revolutionary to discover that the body produces its own morphine-like substances and the body can *learn* to produce them. This knowledge gave control back to the patient suffering from chronic pain.

Stress is an obvious negative factor for the body. Anything that produces stress actually enhances pain; any modality that *lessens* stress *reduces* pain. The pain business all of a sudden took on new life. Mechanisms that "close the gate," like TENS units, were developed to alter the pain. Acupuncture probably works this way, too, by inhibiting the transmission of pain messages. The new understanding of pain transmission physiology also shifted responsibility for pain management over to the patient. If a pain-sufferer could learn ways to increase endorphin levels, pain could be alleviated.

The secret to relief from pain seems to rest with the reduction of chemicals like substance "P" and an increase of substances like endorphins. Before these understandings, all the PWCP had going for him or her was "pain pills," needles, and multiple surgeries. With the advent of new theories, a definite ray of hope broke through—a cloud with a silver lining.

# The Nonphysical Pain Disorder

▲   The *Diagnostic and Statistical Manual of Mental Disorders* or *DSM-III-R* (the "bible" that psychiatrists live by) defines a specific type of pain formally known as *somatoform pain disorder.* Here are the criteria for this diagnosis: (a) the patient must be preoccupied with pain for at least six months, and (b) by an exclusionary process (usually multiple, thorough medical workups), no organic pathology can be demonstrated to justify the experienced pain or the pain is grossly in excess of what would normally be anticipated with the patient's physical findings. In other words, the patient is suffering from severe, prolonged pain that can't be adequately explained.

Women are diagnosed with somatoform pain disorder twice as often as men. There also seems to be an inverse relationship with financial status—the higher up the monetary, socio-economic ladder, the less likely the diagnosis of somatoform pain disorder. Age is not an outstanding characteristic, but the onset of the pain seems to peak in the patient's thirties and forties. Nowhere in the *DSM-III-R* description of this disorder does it infer that the pain experienced is not real. There is simply no medical explanation for the patient's pain.

There are several different ways this disorder has been explained:

1. The *psycho-dynamic* view is that the patient's pain represents an unconscious desire for care and affection. The pain may be a sort of maternal subconscious outreach situation. Another view is that the patient may somehow equate pain with just desserts. Pain is a just punishment for some unpardonable crime or sin. The pain has become intimately interwoven with guilt associated with some transgression, whether factual or imagined.

2. The *behavioral* view is based on a reward premise. Certain pain behavior is rewarded by gains such as not having to work, being comforted, or being looked after, pampered, waited on, or commiserated with. There is also a classic model with this view that associates the pain with pleasurable circumstances. In this model, the pain may be related to being able to stay in the bedroom, being "sick," or being "nursed." Pain is equated with a safe, comfortable place.

3. The *interpersonal* view explains somatoform pain as a way to manipulate others, in much the same way that people with money or power wield influence. Pain is used like a whip, a club, or a sword in order to control others.

4. The *neuro-physiologic* view is based strictly on the biological fact that neurotransmitters mediate pain, and that specifically serotonins and endorphins lower cortical pathway inhibition (as discussed in the last chapter with the Gate theory) and therefore modify pain. Inhibitory fibers carry impulses from the brain and alter pain. Parenthetically, this explanation for somatoform pain makes the most practical sense. We know that anything which enhances endorphin activity or anything that

boosts serotonin levels seems to play a major role in pain management.

## Organic or Somatoform?

Unfortunately, there is no absolute way to differentiate between pain that is organic (from physical causes) or somatoform (from nonphysical causes). There are, however, some strong indications. Organic pain tends to fluctuate, depending on what is going on in your life. So-called "real" pain is influenced by your emotions and any distractions (TV, reading, or a change in focus); it tends to wax and wane. Arthritis is one example. The pain can be terrible at times, and less intense at other times. It will come and go. The pain is chronic and very real, but it has sporadic episodes of flaring up. Somatoform pain, on the other hand, tends to be chronic and *constant.* There's also much more preoccupation with the pain. You may seek out surgery and medical management through pain injections, pills, and other forms of treatment until they become a way of life for you. With somatoform pain there is a greater incidence of alcohol/drug abuse and addiction. Depression is almost always present in cases of somatoform pain. Major depression is supposed to occur in at least 25 to 50% of somatoform pain disorders; minor depression is present in 60 to 100% of the cases.

There are three definite personalities or "types" associated with somatoform pain disorder:

1. *Pain-prone* personalities tend to wallow in their guilt. They are permanently pessimistic. They feel they do not deserve to be happy. They seem to go from one defeat to the next, and they make a career of being "dumped on."

2. *Alexithymic* people tend to be robots. They display little or no emotion. They think mechanically

and literally, have little imagination, and have absolutely no insight. They're absolutely rigid, and there's no give to them. They tend to think that what they don't know isn't worth knowing. They tend to get nowhere in life and are extremely difficult to treat.

3. *Counter-dependent* personalities are those who were super-everything before the pain, and in the post-trauma period they do a complete reversal. They go from being self-reliant, independent, conscientious workaholics to an almost invalid status. They deteriorate into a near infantile state.

## Treatment

Of those who meet the criteria for somatoform pain disorder, people with multiple pre-existing character defects have the poorest prognosis. The deeper into the hole, the harder the climb out. The more baggage, the harder the journey. *Passive,* dependent people do poorly; on the other hand, *aggressive* people, those who are willing to work, do very well. The longer the duration of pain, the worse the prognosis, too. The worse the drug addiction, the worse the prognosis. The better the financial remuneration for "staying sick," the worse the chances of getting well.

What is the treatment for somatoform pain disorder? First, there's no cure—it's yet another manifestation of chronic benign intractable pain. The patient must learn to live with this condition. The pain diminishes, but usually never goes away. Sometimes antidepressants help, but sedative drugs, such as tranquilizers, pain pills, sleeping medications or alcohol, are a disaster for these PWCPs. People with this disorder do much better in groups than in one-to-one therapy. They really need support from others who have the same problem. They need to unburden themselves, share their triumphs and defeats, and get completely honest. They need a supportive program they can sink their teeth into, something with a "can do," "get well" philosophy they can depend on. They would do wonderfully well in a Chronic Pain Anonymous group, a support program for PWCPs that will be outlined in greater detail later in this book.

# Profile of a PWCP

▲   When pain starts to rule your life, it means that you have lost control. When a person addicted to a drug (alcohol, cocaine, heroin, marijuana, pain pills, tranquilizers, etc.) gets out of control, it results in terrible trouble. When your life is out of control, it brings about a great deal of misery. It can destroy your home, social, and work life. When pain erodes your life in any way, shape, or form, it's time to ask for help. In profiling the life of a PWCP (a Person With Chronic Pain), there are several prime characteristics that signal the need for help.

## Loss of Control

*Loss of control* is a prime characteristic of the PWCP, and it is often cited in discussions about alcoholics. You do not have a problem with alcohol, for instance, if you are able to drink with impunity. If you are able to walk away from the bar when you have had "enough"—and do that for a lifetime—it does not result in trouble. Alcoholics do not walk away, and the result is a progressive and often fatal disease. If a PWCP sees his or her life falling apart "because of the pain," it's reasonable to assume they are no longer in control.

If pain severely interferes with a PWCP's personal relationships, like between a husband and wife, parent and child, or significant others, then it's time to take corrective action. When pain destroys intimacy and sexual relations, it naturally results in serious trouble. There are many ways chronic pain can progressively destroy any semblance of family life: a sour disposition, morose outlook on life, severe restrictions in routine family functions, lack of interest in loved ones, open hostility, bitterness, financial woes, disheveled appearance, egocentricity, severe restriction of mobility, drug abuse or addiction, self-pity, cynical attitude, inability to sleep, and depression. When the presence of pain causes any significant dysfunction, the end result is civil war on the home front, and the home is left in shambles. When this loss of control happens to any PWCP, they need to seek help.

All too often there is little or no social life left for a person suffering from chronic pain. Pain has a way of snuffing out your social life. People quickly tire of your usual litany of complaints. The pain makes you miserable and it invariably causes you to lash out at others, driving them away. Friends disappear. Pain obviously limits your activity, and your interests begin to dwindle. In this day and age, the omnipresent television often becomes the PWCP's best friend. Social activities demanding any physical participation become a long-gone pleasure. Hiking, bowling, golf, tennis, swimming, boating, fishing, hunting, dancing, parties, or church activities become physically unmanageable. It's not unusual to see vivacious, interesting, intelligent people withdraw into shells, and as time passes, they bear little resemblance to their former selves. When you are in control, these things do not happen. If a PWCP can rise above the pain and not allow it to interfere with social activities, then he or she is indeed still in control. Few patients with chronic pain seem to find themselves in this position, however. They experience many personal losses, but they are still social beings, and they need to interact with other people. The loss of a social life tends to leave a huge hole in a PWCP's life.

The routine of a job forces people into your life, and doing good work gives you a feeling of peace and accomplishment. After a hard day's work you can sleep well because, most of the time, you are mentally or physically worn out. If you work to the best of your ability, you will usually be satisfied with yourself—and that adds to your feelings of self-worth. It's been said that the most aggressive threat that can be thrown at a good worker is the loss of a job. Your paycheck is a well-deserved reward for labor, but the loss of your paycheck would make you feel unsuccessful and unproductive. When a person can no longer function on the job because of pain, the PWCP suffers yet another personal tragedy. There is the loss of a regular paycheck to cope with, and little joy living on a reduced income. The PWCP has little self-respect sitting around all day doing nothing but coping with pain. Chronic pain sufferers often lose their ability to work, but if they can rise above the pain and maintain their employment by learning to cope (and therefore manage), there is no need for special intervention or help.  When pain results in the loss of meaningful work, however, it often pushes the PWCP to the depths of despair. Many suicides can be blamed on the loss of an occupation. The PWCP's ambitions, dreams, hopes, and financial security are often completely lost due to chronic pain—and it's a bitter pill to swallow, yet another form of losing control.

## Preoccupation

If pain becomes the "center of the universe," it spells nothing but trouble. When every waking moment is consumed with thoughts of pain, the PWCP needs help. *Preoccupation* with pain is another prime characteristic of the PWCP, and when a person's life revolves around pain, it's no longer "normal." The PWCP may develop daily plans around a series of pain medications, and here again, the alcoholic model can illustrate that something is very wrong. An alcoholic usually can't do anything *without* alcohol. Every date, meeting, sports activity, or social function becomes an opportunity to drink. The first question is always, "Who's going to bring the booze?" An alcoholic gets up in the morning and goes to bed at night thinking about alcohol, and life revolves around a drug. Similarly, when a patient suffering from chronic pain becomes preoccupied with pain, when every plan, every action, and every future move is predicated on pain, it's time to seek help.

On the beach at Anzio in World War II, it was documented that there was only negligible use of narcotics on wounded soldiers during the landing. Soldiers missing arms and legs did not complain of pain. Bombs were bursting nearby, bullets were whistling over their heads, the noise was hellish, and many of the wounded spent hours without any pain medication—and they asked for none. They were too busy trying to stay alive. They were focused on survival. But when the crisis subsided, the pain descended with a vengeance. The mind obviously plays a huge part in how pain is perceived in the body. If the PWCP can divert focus away from the pain, it helps enormously. On the other hand, when someone is preoccupied with pain, it's bound to get worse. The PWCP has to learn to stop the preoccupation, but that's easier said than done. Preoccupation is a major characteristic of anyone suffering from chronic pain.

## Adverse Consequences

People who suffer from benign intractable pain aren't stupid. They know that the pain is eroding their lives. When they take an honest inventory of themselves, they realize that pain is severely interfering with their home, work, and social life. They see the need for change, and they know deep in their hearts that *they* need to change. They know that their lives are being ruined by the burden of pain they carry, but they continue the same destructive conduct. No matter what the *adverse consequences,* the PWCP's behavior change goes in a negative direction.

Here again, there is a similarity between the PWCP and the drug addict. A drug addict knows the path he or she is taking is a lonely spiral into oblivion, yet there is oftentimes no effort made to alter the course. An alcoholic knows that booze will eventually kill and everything will be lost in the process, but the conduct is unaltered. Continued use in spite of adverse consequences is characteristic of addiction. It's also characteristic of a person with chronic benign intractable pain. PWCPs typically allow the pain to grind them into a shell of their former selves. It's not that they don't know better, and it's not that they are lacking any intelligence. They simply are not able to change...very much like the addict.

Change comes from within, and no one can make the necessary changes for another. People who are able to make positive changes can take a deserved bow; certainly those who do not go on taking more beatings. People who suffer chronic benign intractable pain never become 100% pain-free, but by taking charge of themselves, by assuming command, and by accepting responsibility, they can learn to cope with life on its own terms and decrease the magnitude of their pain. Alcoholics do not stay sober by accident; they work at it. When they quit working at it, they relapse. The PWCP has to learn everything possible about what will produce positive change and then go after it like his or her life depends upon it. And their lives often do depend on it.

## Denial

PWCPs are generally full of *denial.* It's a powerful defense mechanism, and the PWCP typically enlists most of the mental defense mechanisms, almost without fail. Patients with chronic pain delude themselves all the time:

• "Yes, the pain is bad. It's terrible, but I'm coping with it!"

• "Sure, pain has incapacitated me, but I don't let it interfere with my life!"

• "It hasn't hurt *my* home, work, or social life!"

• "I know I take too many pain pills, but I'm still in control!"

• "I can stop the pain pills anytime I want!"

• "What the hell!"

• "You think I can't do without sleeping pills and tranquilizers?"

• "So, I've had five back surgeries; the next one will take away my pain!"

• "I've had headaches for thirty years, but it's only a matter of time before a medical miracle will come along. Then I'll stop the narcotics and tranquilizers!"

• "I've seen fifteen different doctors, but I just heard about a fantastic doctor in Podunk, Iowa!"

These are all statements typical of PWCPs in a state of denial.

## Rationalization

*Rationalization* is another black-belt form of mental defense mechanism. It seems that the sharper the patient, the more excuses they invent to continue their harmful conduct. Perhaps any bizarre conduct can be excused if the PWCP works at it hard enough, and it's true that most people can talk themselves into just about anything they really want. The PWCP usually hammers negative behavior into something that conveniently fits into their agenda. (The realization that the hole is round and the peg is square is incidental.) Rationalization allows the PWCP to live with themselves in comfort. It often takes a group setting or an outside third party to get through the rationalization defense. Many PWCPs go through life insisting white is black. Some chronic pain sufferers are stubborn and bull-headed, convincing themselves that there's a good reason for their behavior. Rationalization, however, blocks the PWCP's progress and allows destructive habits to continue. And it's a poor reason for someone to die.

## Projection

*Projection* is another defense mechanism often used by the PWCP. The patient with chronic pain often finds himself or herself indulging in the misery brought on by pain. Some exude self-pity, as they point a finger of blame at others, usually those who supposedly allow them to continue their destructive behavior. It's the "money-grubbing surgeon, the lousy lawyer, the wife, the kids, the Internal Revenue, the System, the clergy, the President, the insurance racket, the sick society, crime in the streets," or anything else. Projection doesn't exactly sparkle with good mental health, and it takes the PWCP's focus off of themselves and away from taking personal responsibility for pain management and self-improvement.

## Repression and Suppression

*Repression* is another characteristic of the person with chronic pain. Repression allows PWCPs to bury in their subconscious what they don't want to deal with. People with chronic benign intractable pain quite often end up refusing to deal with facts, figures, or everyday reality. They just submerge everything in the subconscious and let it sit there. When this repression process is done intentionally, another label is put on it—*suppression.* Repression and suppression tend to keep a person sick. Not dealing with issues doesn't make them disappear. Alcoholics Anonymous has a saying that "a person is as sick as his secrets." It essentially means that the "garbage" that accumulates in a person's head must be thrown out periodically. The attic must be swept clean and it must stay clean (at least giving it a focused try!) if a person is to enjoy good mental health. Good mental health reduces pain; it doesn't take the pain away, but it makes it so that the PWCP can at least live with it, without it eating them alive.

## The PWCP and Addiction

Is there such a thing as a "typical" chronic pain profile? If there is, it's very difficult to pinpoint. In working with chronic pain, as with addictions, all you can do is examine how someone's suffering is getting in the way of a healthy life. The pain is a constant, underlying condition, but it's often masked by many unhealthy behaviors. If that's the case, then it's time for the PWCP to do something about the suffering. Millions of people in the United States (and many other millions worldwide) experience chronic benign intractable pain and their lives are altered so significantly that they have little choice but to seek help. The alternative is a dismal future with little or nothing to look forward to except constant pain. If a person has pain for over six months, the chances are somewhere between great and overwhelming that it has become locked in their central nervous system for good. Thereafter, the pain feeds on itself and all the PWCP can do is learn to live with it. The lucky people who can rise above the pain without it adversely affecting their lives don't need special help beyond that which keeps them on their path of self-help and pain management. If something works, why fix it? These people are, however, the fortunate few.

In addictionology, much time is spent trying to convince people they need help. Sometimes the only thing that will get an addict into treatment, or even into a position where they realize they need help, is through an intervention. The intervention process involves people who are willing to take a risk, usually those who care the most. Some addicts never seem to get the message unless an intervention takes place. The addict often doesn't even have a clue how their lives are affected and how their behavior is harming those who love them. An intervention provides an opportunity for those who have not yet been driven off to come together and present reality therapy to the one who is suffering. The process rarely fails.

With chronic benign intractable pain, professionals often see the same addictive patterns and the same lack of insight. It often takes an intervention in order to get the patient to get help. It takes those who really care and love the PWCP to get involved and get their attention. Chronic pain sufferers, like addicts, can get to be experts at ignoring their circumstances.

At times, reality floats in and out of their awareness, but the PWCP usually learns to use defense mechanisms better than a chess master uses pawns. Unless those who care can get through to the PWCP, conditions will worsen. The self-destructive conduct will continue, dragging other family members down with them. Family members, friends, and loved ones may end up paying and paying and paying.

Years ago, healthcare professionals came up with profiles for the addictive personality. The profiles were interesting subject matter, but they proved to be of little clinical or practical value. Their bottom line was that addiction is characterized by loss of control, preoccupation, continued use of substances despite adverse consequences, and distorted thinking (notably denial). Genetic, psychosocial, and environmental factors influence the development and manifestation of addictions.

Similar to the addiction model, people with chronic benign intractable pain are also characterized by loss of control, preoccupation, continued detrimental behavior despite adverse consequences, and distorted thinking (notably denial). It may not at all be genetic in origin, but psychosocial and environmental factors influence the development and manifestation of problems plaguing the PWCP.

## The Key Development Factors

The psychosocial factors in chronic benign intractable pain are profound. Very few challenge the fact that the mind influences pain. Often, however, well-meaning people will think poorly of people with chronic pain. Because you cannot objectively see the pain in others, because pain impulses produced by the original tissue trauma have long ceased, because nothing can be definitely shown to cause the pain, you might think the pain is "all in the head!" The PWCP is not a "nut case," however—their pain is real and constant. People who have chronic benign intractable pain are all quite sane. You can be mentally ill and have chronic pain, just as any mental health patient may also be addicted to alcohol or any legal or illicit drug. For the most part, PWCPs have "normal" mental functioning. Most PWCPs readily admit that at times they *fear* for their sanity when the pain gets out of hand, but generally most keep their balance, despite their monumental problem. Physicians who specialize in pain management acknowledge this fact and frankly are outraged when charges are made against PWCPs, like "the pain is imaginary!", "All she needs is a hobby!", or "You don't know what real pain is!" The pain you would experience as a PWCP is as real as if you just had a leg chopped off.

This chapter has already addressed the social side of the psychosocial factors which are part of the PWCP's life. Chronic pain severely restricts social activities to the point of driving everyone away. As social beings, this can lead to profound depression. When the TV becomes your only source of contact with the outside world, something is very wrong. When you change from an outgoing, lively person into a hypersensitive recluse, someone should intervene before it's too late. The PWCP (and everyone else!) needs people in his/her life, and chronic benign intractable pain is famous for shoving them away.

Environmental factors also influence the development and manifestations of chronic pain. Pain wasn't even noticed on the beach at Anzio, and slightly-built mothers have lifted cars to rescue their children at the scene of an accident. When enough adrenaline rushes into your system, you can do amazing things. When the focus shifts away from the pain to another subject of attention, you will experience less pain.

A non-stressful, peaceful environment also does wonders for people suffering from chronic benign intractable pain. Unfortunately, the PWCP does not live in a non-stressful, peaceful world, and they evidently weren't placed on earth to live as Mary Poppins. Life is full of demands and stress, and pain will get worse in a hostile, stressful environment (unless survival becomes your complete preoccupation). If you are in constant pain, you don't need additional stress. You need to learn how to deal with the stress coming into your life with better efficiency. Incidentally, stress is not all bad! Without stress, the chances are that people would all run around with the alacrity of an amoeba. Any way you can learn to reduce or alleviate stress will help ease pain, however. Your surroundings play a large part in pain reduction, and here are several factors to be concerned about:

- Raw nerves
- Anxiety
- Turmoil
- Living with people who have a defeatist attitude
- Living with people who wait on you because of your pain
- Living with someone who discourages physical exercise
- Living with someone who encourages obesity
- The use of drugs
- Physicians who prescribe just about anything

These and other environmental factors are crucial when it comes to influencing the development and manifestations of chronic pain.

The role genetic factors play in the PWCP's profile is still being studied. People certainly inherit the ability to feel pain, and they genetically inherit certain predispositions. "Blue collar" workers who perform heavy physical labor fare better with pain tolerance when compared to "white collar" workers who are often unwilling to put up with physical discomfort. A miner or a longshoreman/woman is likely to shrug off injuries that would incapacitate an office worker.

In certain cultures, showing pain is discouraged. The traditional Native American cultures, for instance, were famous for stoicism. Allowing an enemy to witness your suffering was to lose face. The Spartans also suffered in silence. Were these traits genetic or environmental in origin? The same nervous system has been passed on to all human beings, yet there is diversity in the ways pain is expressed. This has led to many stereotypes, like the saying "the Irish drink because they love to suffer; Jews don't drink because it interferes with their suffering." Historically, certain races have become noted for their ability to accept pain, and classes within a society seem to be able to bear pain better than others.

Genetic, environmental, and psychosocial factors are all involved in the manifestation and development of chronic benign intractable pain. All of these influence your perception of pain. Your nervous system is inherited, and not all systems are the same from person to person. Minor trauma to you may result in excruciating pain to another. "Hypersensitive nervous systems" are inherited.

In the field of pain physiology, it's difficult to separate the key genetic factors from the environmental ones, but this whole subject will be fascinating research for future generations. Again, the more information unearthed about the origins of pain and how pain signals are transmitted in the body, the more tools you'll have for pain management. Literally every angle of pain physiology should be explored. In the next chapter, you'll see how the medical profession has tried to help the PWCP cope with and manage the everyday reality of chronic pain.

# Medical "Solutions"

▲   Do you know the difference between minor and major surgery? Minor surgery is a procedure that is done on someone else; major surgery is any procedure done on *you.*

Surgery and other medical procedures are really no laughing matter, and they are of key importance to a PWCP. Modern medicine has provided people with a plethora of surgical and other invasive procedures to eliminate or alleviate pain. It's typical of most patients who have chronic benign intractable pain to have been subjected to many "cures" by any number of sincere physicians or other ancillary medical practitioners. It's not unusual to see patients in chronic pain management units with a history of five to twenty-five major surgeries, plus experience with every modality, electrical or chemical, known to the mainstream of medicine. All of these PWCPs seem to have one thing in common. They still have their pain.

There are many medical disciplines out there, all claiming to rid the patient of pain. Every medical advocate is convinced that their discipline will do the trick. Would that it were true! Even within their own disciplines, many individuals are thoroughly convinced they hold all the answers and others in the field are either ignorant or second-rate. The success of a modality often depends on how it's delivered. When a service is delivered with unwavering certitude, it's much more likely to succeed. When people act like what they don't know already isn't worth knowing, their treatments are more likely to work, and some people in the pain business are terrific sales people.

Most of the professionals who deliver service to the patient with chronic pain have *some* success. Despite all the modern miracles in medicine, however, chronic pain remains an enigma. One of the raging arguments is whether the focus of treatment should be physiological or psychological, and there seems to be no one answer. The consensus is that it should be multidimensional, and a part of this multidisciplinary approach may turn out to be invasive procedures. "Invasive" connotes needles and surgery, procedures that "invade" the body. Let's look at the most common of these.

## Needles

Most "needle jockeys" are anesthesiologists, specially trained physicians who put people to sleep for operations. Some anesthesiologists go into specialized training in order to provide a service termed "neural blockage." It may be used as a diagnostic or therapeutic procedure, and it's used in a variety of pain problems. When used therapeutically, a local anesthetic, either by itself or in combination with a steroid, is injected into a specific place in the body. Most of these procedures are performed on an outpatient basis.

*Sphenopalatine ganglion blocks* are used for the management of acute migraines, acute cluster headaches, and several other neuralgias.

*Stellate ganglion blocks* are used for conditions known as reflex sympathetic dystrophy of the face, neck, and upper thorax; sympathetically mediated malignant pain; and also in herpes zoster.

*Celiac plexus block* is used as a diagnostic tool as well as a prognostic indicator for the relief of chronic pancreatitis pain or cancer pain in the upper abdominal region.

*Lumbar sympathetic nerve blocks* are frequently employed as a diagnostic maneuver for sympathetic dystrophy of the lower leg, specifically to see if the blood supply is improved and/or to relieve pain. It's also used to treat cases where the blood supply needs to be improved in the extremities for people with frostbite or herpes zoster.

*Occipital nerve blocks* relieve occipital neuralgia.

*Epidural nerve blocks* are used extensively in the diagnosis and treatment of many pain syndromes. They are prescribed to relieve pain in the neck, chest, and low back (particularly radiculopathy, where the pain radiates into the buttocks and legs). As you might expect, these blocks are a treatment for herpes zoster, low back sprains, reflex sympathetic dystrophy, vascular insufficiency, and frostbite.

*Cervical epidural nerve blocks* have been used to treat long-term tension headaches, "whiplash" type injuries, and severe fibromyalgia.

*Trigeminal nerve blocks* are used as an adjunct with other more specific medications for relief of facial pain.

Local, more superficial injections are used to relieve pain syndromes of the head and neck. Discreet hypersensitive areas, called myofascial trigger points, are first palpated (felt with the fingers) in the musculature of the head, neck, and trapezius muscles and then injected with a local anesthesia, often in combination with a steroid.

*Intercostal nerve blocks* are performed for rib fractures or post surgical lung removals or chest tubes. Catheters are sometimes placed between the layers of the pleura to relieve acute and chronic pain in the chest.

There are many chronic pain management outpatient clinics that specialize in most of these nerve blocks, but they also integrate multidisciplinary approaches such as exercise physiology, TENS units, counseling, biofeedback, guided imagery, etc. The primary emphasis, however, is the needle, and the physicians doing the injecting do not work for minimum wage. They are sold on the concept that nociceptive input is present in the periphery or autonomic nervous system and they can stop it. People are certainly drawn to this concept because it means someone is going to take the pain away for good. There is little doubt that it is efficacious in an acute pain situation; chronic pain, of course, is very different. If you buy into chronic pain being nothing other than extended acute pain, the philosophy fits quite well.

## Surgical Procedures

Neurosurgeons are trained to do radical surgery to alleviate cancer pain. They remove nerves (*peripheral neurectomies*), when indicated. Invasive tumors often put pressure on nerves which sometimes causes excruciating pain. This is particularly true in the area of the ribs. People with recurrent cancer of the rectum or bladder, with perineal or genital pain, require an *alcohol rhizotomy* or an *alcohol spinal.* Instead of cutting the nerve (a *rhizotomy*), alcohol chemically destroys the nerve just outside the cord. The rhizotomy is obviously a limited procedure.

Another procedure, called a *commissural*

*myelotomy,* is used occasionally for the relief of bilateral pelvic pain. The spinal cord is sectioned, severing the nerves which ascend through the spinal cord to the thalamus. The procedure, however, has many drawbacks.

Another operation, a *medullary tractotomy,* requires sectioning of the descending tract of the trigeminal nerves in the lower medulla to provide relief for a painful unilateral lesion of the head and neck. Cerebral operations are still being performed for relief of pain, but only in selective areas usually involving frontal fibers. In the United States the climate is somewhat hostile to such "psychosurgery."

A *cordotomy* involves the sectioning of the spinothalamic tract of the spinal cord on the side opposite the patient's pain site. It's usually employed for cancer pain. It's a formidable procedure, particularly if the pain is bilateral.

*Hypophysectomy* is most often performed to relieve pain from cancer of the breast and of the prostate, when metastasized. Hypophysectomy means that the pituitary is either cut out or destroyed chemically or eradicated by a radio-frequency probe.

Another surgical procedure involves electrodes planted in the brain to relieve pain. The electrodes seem to work by stimulating certain portions of the brain to produce endorphins.

*Spinal opiates* have been used with great promise in alleviating chronic cancer pain. Surgeons install a catheter in the epidural space in the spine, and then morphine can be injected directly where it can do the most good, usually every six to twelve hours. Obviously this technique is generally used in the lower spine region since higher level applications may cause respiratory depression.

Surgery has also been used for trigeminal neuralgia, a disorder of the fifth cranial nerve which produces bouts of severe, seconds-long lancinating pain (most often throughout the upper jaw or side of the face). The surgical approaches include a cutting of the trigeminal root or destroying the nerve electrically or chemically.

## TENS Units

Drs. Ronald Melzak and Patrick Wall are responsible for the modern basis of the electro-medical treatment of pain. In 1965, they proposed the theory that hypothetical "gates" in the dorsal root could be closed and therefore block pain. The gate is positioned where the large "A" fibers and the slower "C" pain fibers carry pain impulses into the central nervous system. C. Norman Shealy, M.D., a neurosurgeon and an illustrious pioneer in the pain management field, began surgically implanting dorsal column stimulators based on this principle.

*Dorsal column stimulation* was primarily used for the relief of intense chronic back pain. It was speculated that stimulation of the dorsal columns of the spinal cord, at about the level of the pain, would stop the pain. Electrodes were placed, usually by a neurosurgeon, on a peripheral nerve of the dorsal column. They were connected to a radio receiver implanted under the skin. The receiver was activated by an external transmitter attached to a coupling antenna. After a wave of enthusiasm in the 1970s, this treatment dropped out of sight when the promising early results could not be reliably reproduced. Some neurosurgeons still use it, but controversy surrounds the overall use of implanted electrodes.

TENS Units (Transcutaneous Electrical Nerve Stimulators) were later found to be as effective as the dorsal column stimulators. Shealy discovered that devices that transmit electricity outside the skin were just as effective as dorsal column stimulation, without the risk of surgery. Shealy's work started the widespread use of TENS Units, which were first commercially developed in 1967 by Medtronic and StimTec. About 200,000 TENS Units were prescribed by physicians in 1991.

Mechanically, a TENS Unit device selectively dispenses electricity from a small box a little larger than a pack of cigarettes, usually clipped to a belt or other article of clothing. The patient administers his or her own dose of electricity from this highly portable mini machine. Most TENS Units work under the 400 micro-second range, and they are powered by alkaline batteries, often rechargeable. Self-adhesive, disposable synthetic electrodes are used.

The principle of the TENS Unit is simple enough. The unit stimulates the "A" fibers and they compete with the "C" pain fibers. When all the impulses terminate in the same area of the spinal cord, the "gate" is closed. Something similar probably happens with the pain relief from ice, heat, stretching, and manipulation.

A TENS Unit operates under several variables. The pulse repetition rate setting on each unit delivers frequency. The lower the setting, the greater the frequency, and the greater the potential to relieve pain. (Endorphin release has been demonstrated at low PRR settings.) People usually start out on the lowest pulse repetition rate. Pulse width spreads the current. The further apart the electrodes, the wider the pulse width should be. Electrode placement is quite variable. The area of pain is sort of "squeezed" or "sandwiched" between the electrodes.

TENS Units have been used for headaches, phantom limb pain, arthritis, post-op pain, low back pain, radiculopathy (a disturbance of function or pathological change in one or more of the nerve roots), cancer pain, angina, dysmenorrhea (painful menstruation), visceral pain, herpes zoster neuralgia—just about every type of pain. About the only contraindication is when a patient has a pacemaker or is pregnant. Use of a unit on the head and neck is watched with caution, and use around heavy machinery can be a concern.

One of the problems with the TENS unit is that it requires a good deal of knowledge and understanding to operate it. Results have not been uniform. One of the reasons for the inconsistent results from individual to individual is that so often the TENS Unit is prescribed for patient use with little or no instruction. Wave form, pulse repetition rate, intensity, current (alternating or direct), treatment time, and electrode placement all have to be factored into the pain equation, and that can be confusing. People have to be educated and their progress monitored for a TENS Unit to be effective.

It's often difficult with the TENS Unit to find the right combination of variables to bring relief. Many professionals just toss the unit to the patient with instructions to "try it out!" It may not be perfect, but "any port in a storm." TENS is definitely one of the most reasonable pain-relief devices on the current scene. Properly applied, it has helped many people. There are a number of individuals, however, who experience relief for a short period before becoming tolerant to the unit—and then the pain returns. (There is no current explanation as to why people develop that tolerance factor to the TENS Unit.) If you buy a unit, you will be stuck with it, and such units are quite expensive. Make certain a unit provides you some relief on an ongoing basis by renting one before you make a substantial investment you may regret later.

# Drugs and the PWCP

▲   It seems that the *majority* of patients with
chronic benign intractable pain become hooked on
one or more drugs. Alcohol is, of course, a drug, and
some PWCPs retreat into a bottle. A large percentage
of them end up addicted to combinations of narcotics, tranquilizers, sleeping pills, alcohol, or other
mind-altering substances. Drugs become a way to
cope with the pain.

By definition, "intractable" means just that—the
pain doesn't go away. "Benign" distinguishes this
type of pain from "malignant" (which is cancer), so by
comparison, this pain is more "favorable," "not so
bad," and "beneficial" (obviously it's a misnomer).
Chronic benign intractable pain, by definition, is
non-cancerous or non-malignant pain that simply
doesn't go way.

When earlier chapters reviewed the physiology of
pain, you learned that when end organs or specialized pain receptors (nociceptors) are stimulated, a
pain message is sent to the brain. It's transmitted by
an intricate network of nerves connected by syn-
apses. Neurotransmitters carry the impulse between
nerve endings. The brain and the spinal cord are the
central nervous system (CNS), through which the

impulse is relayed. The brain interprets the message and responds accordingly. Along the path of transmission, many interesting things happen. Interconnections take place that short-circuit the message in the CNS, and a pain response is made through the nervous system in any number of places in the body. This is a quick rundown of how acute pain works, but the problem emerges when acute pain turns into sub-acute, and finally chronic benign intractable pain. When pain gets locked up in the CNS, the chances are quite poor that it will ever subside. A leading theory among specialists in pain management is that pain turns into a self-feeding mechanism, not unlike a perpetual motion machine. Once that happens, the PWCP is stuck with it—it's a life sentence, as surely as if a judge bangs the gavel and hands down the decision.

## Problems in the Making

Physicians deal with acute pain quite well. All doctors are quite capable of pulling out their trusty prescription pads and writing for medications which take away, or at least placate, their patients' pain. If anything, most err in prescribing too little medication when acute pain is an issue. In a week or so, the pain is much better or often gone for most patients. Physicians usually start by prescribing weak analgesics, depending on their judgment. Remember, acute pain lasts less than one month, but drugs become a concern in the sub-acute stage. Narcotics continued into the sub-acute period carry addiction potential. If the patient develops a tolerance to the medication, it means that more and more drugs are needed to achieve the old result. Also, if narcotics are stopped, withdrawal symptoms will surface. Mild symptoms are quite common, and these include tremors, weakness, sweating, hyper-reflexia, and gastrointestinal illness. Major symptoms of physical withdrawal, if they occur, can become very serious. Invariably, when physical withdrawal takes place, pain results. All drug addicts or people going through withdrawal experience pain, restlessness, agitation, muscle cramps, "goose bumps," runny nose and eyes, anorexia, pinpoint pupils, headaches, and sleeplessness. Withdrawal signs typically appear in four to six hours. Demerol withdrawal generally peaks in ten to twelve hours, heroin in thirty-six hours, and methadone in about three days.

Surgical procedures present special problems. Surgeons have a duty to keep a patient as pain-free as possible, but not forever. Surgeons have a tendency to use narcotics aggressively for several weeks and then send the patient back to the referring physician who sometimes keeps filling the prescriptions. Many post-surgical patients are willing to put up with very little discomfort and they overdo their use of medications. If the pills are around, they take them and soon ask for more. Some people do have a low tolerance for pain. The pendulum may swing the other way, too, and many patients will put up with awful pain and never ask for anything. As the nociceptive input subsides, so should the pain. The problem is, quite often, it doesn't.

When prescribing drugs, surgeons can only judge on what their experience and their "gut feelings" dictate. This is true for anyone who is qualified to write for drugs—they guess a lot. Probably most surgeons under-prescribe for pain in the acute phase, but unfortunately make up for it by giving much too much analgesic in the sub-acute and chronic phases. One principle that seems to escape many physicians is that as a patient becomes hooked on drugs, withdrawal symptoms occur, and when that happens, patients experience pain. Many patients take narcotics for months and years because they can't face the withdrawal. As soon as they start developing any withdrawal symptoms, they take more pills to "cure" their problem. Of course, it means a lifetime of narcotics with all the turmoil involved in acquiring them. Sooner or later, even the most liberal physician cuts off the patient's supply. At that time the "Doctor Hopper" syndrome sets in. The patient has to find three to four new "candy men/women." The drug problem can escalate to be frightfully expensive and dangerous. And John Law takes a dim view of forging prescriptions or buying narcotics on the street.

## Benzodiazepines

Narcotics are just one of the pill problems. Invariably, PWCPs become very anxious and depressed. Physicians swiftly dispose of anxiety by prescribing the tranquilizer of the month, ordinarily a benzodiazepine. The original benzodiazepine was librium, then valium, followed by ativan, and then xanax. Many other benzodiazepines have come and gone, but they are all related. Through the years, most "newly discovered" benzodiazepines have become shorter acting, and all of them are bears when it comes to withdrawal. With almost twenty-five years in the addiction field, the author feels the withdrawal from benzodiazepines is the worst, without exception. Heroin is a "piece of cake" compared to benzodiazepines. Not *all* PWCPs go the tranquilizer route, just *most.*

The majority of physicians are very aware that the mighty prescription pad relieves tension. Mention "nerves" and the reflex is the written prescription.

Probably four or five pharmaceutical salespeople have visited that physician the same week extolling the benefits of their "tension relieving" medication. And people show up at the doctor's office *expecting* a prescription. If a physician refuses to write for a tranquilizer, the chances are pretty good it will end the relationship. At that stage in the process, the person with chronic pain just moves on to another physician.

Pain, obviously, leads to a terrific amount of tension. If you have anxiety, it's perfectly justified to take anxiolytic (anxiety-relieving) medication. You as the patient think so, the physician thinks so, certainly the psychiatrist thinks so and, of course, the general public thinks so. Television commercials make it quite clear that we are not supposed to suffer even minor pain. Tension goes away with "Miller Time," sleep comes with any number of medications, and the answers to life's problems come in pill form.

## Sleeping Pills

Sleeping pills are a major problem with PWCPs. People with chronic benign intractable pain have a significant problem with sleep: pain prevents sleep. Falling asleep is tough; staying asleep is even worse. No one ever died from a lack of sleep, but it makes life miserable. Watching reruns on the tube wears thin in a hurry. It's hard to keep a "sunny" disposition on a few hours of sleep every night. The natural thing to do is ask for sleeping pills—and even more benzodiazepines!

Probably the leading cause of insomnia in the United States is sleeping pills, and just behind sleeping pills is alcohol. When sleeping pills are taken for any length of time, physiological and psychological dependence develops. Tolerance is a big factor, too. One pill doesn't work, and soon two and three will not do the job. Eventually, those sweet-looking sleeping pills become a mortal enemy. Sleep patterns become worse than ever. It turns into quite a nightmarish dilemma.

To really get good rest, your body demands Stage IV and REM (rapid eye movement) sleep. When you put your head on the pillow, you gradually enter Stage I, then progress to II, III, and Stage IV sleep. In IV, you are resting blissfully and you experience restorative sleep. You do not stay in Stage IV long before you start coming up, usually progressing from IV to III to II to I, but you don't awaken. You enter into REM sleep. In this stage you dream. You also get wonderful sleep in the REM state. This healthy sleep cycle repeats about every ninety minutes all night long, meaning you go through four or five cycles per night. (All this information, by the way, is well documented by sleep specialists.) Sleeping pills and alcohol rob the PWCP of Stage IV and REM sleep, but if these drugs are off limits, how can the PWCP sleep?

It seems that few people are happy with the accepted recommendations for sleep. PWCPs are no exception. The only difference is that most of them backed into their sleep problems because of their pain. Sleeping pills should be used judiciously *only* for a limited period. The "limited period" is difficult to define. It may be different for every man, woman, or child, and a host of factors must be considered: overall health, age, environment, history, weight, etc. One thing is certain, all soporifics (sleep-inducers) should be prescribed for *brief* periods, days to weeks.

There are positive steps for PWCPs to help them sleep and steer them away from drugs. Exercise is wonderful for good sleep. Everyone sleeps better through relaxation exercises, meditation, guided imagery, being at peace with yourself and others, quiet surroundings, going to bed at the same time every night, eliminating naps, avoiding stimulating beverages, cutting down on coffee and cigarettes, and not obsessing over any of your problems. It helps to move out of the bedroom if sleep doesn't come. Trying *not* to fall asleep is sometimes beneficial. A hot bath before retiring helps. Good sex helps. Anything helps but pills.

Of all the modalities, probably exercise is the most important mechanism as an adjunct to sleep. This is not the best news for a patient suffering from chronic benign intractable pain. When pain is present, exercise is not a priority. Nonetheless, when you are physically worn out, sleep comes easily. Probably the second most important adjunct to sleeping is your state of mind. It's almost impossible to sleep when your mind is fired-up, and pain has a way of doing just that. To be able to relax, to be at peace with the family, to eliminate discord with people on the job and with friends—these things go a long way to induce sleep. Again, anything but pills!

## Antidepressants

Depression is considered the most common emotional disorder associated with chronic pain, and it's said to occur in 5% of the total U.S. population. It's reasonable to assume that depression lowers pain tolerance and contributes to the problem. Depression, reactive to pain, is almost a given. Depression may also precede the pain, but most of the time it's the other way around. The *Diagnostic and Statistical Manual of Mental Disorders* lists a variety of symptoms for depression.

The symptoms for depression include:

1. Poor appetite or significant weight loss (when not dieting), increased appetite, or significant weight gain
2. Insomnia or hypersomnia
3. Psychomotor retardation or agitation
4. Loss of interest in or enjoyment of sex
5. Social withdrawal
6. Feelings of unworthiness, self reproach, or inappropriate guilt
7. Recurrent thoughts of death, suicidal ideation, wishes to be dead, or a suicide attempt
8. Fearfulness or crying

Many "average" people walking the streets would qualify as being depressed, particularly if the person asking the question wants to make it turn out that way. Just about any square peg can be hammered into a round hole with a sledge hammer. In these modern times, it seems that if you are not taking an antidepressant or a like substance, you simply aren't "with it."

PWCPs will sometimes be depressed endogenously, but they'll deny it. "Endogenous" means that the depression develops from within. An antidepressant comes to the rescue by restoring the body's neurotransmitter balance. "Macho" or more assertive people sometimes are significantly depressed but refuse to accept it. Most people who suffer from chronic benign intractable pain are just like other "average" people, but they have to carry around about fifty extra pounds of burden all day because of their pain. If that wouldn't make someone depressed, then nothing would. Antidepressants may also assist with chronic pain treatment because at least in some instances they help alleviate some "neuritic" pain (inflammation of the nerves). Further, addiction to antidepressants is not a problem.

Antidepressants, originally used as an adjunct to psychotherapy, are drugs that may have a promising place in the overall treatment of chronic pain. Since the 1960s, theories involving the depletion or alteration of norepinephrine and serotonin have evolved, and effective antidepressants have surfaced which affect the concentrations of these neurotransmitters. Neurophysiologists discovered that nerves transmit impulses across a microscopic abyss called a synapse. The end of one nerve is termed the presynaptic terminal and the beginning of the new nerve, the postsynaptic. It helps to think about it as a passenger arriving on one train, crossing over the station and boarding another train in order to continue his journey. The "first-line" antidepressants block the re-uptake of norepinephrine, serotonin, or both. (If people arrive at a train station in great numbers with the express purpose of transferring to another train, and they can't get back on the old train, the train station will soon be crowded. An abundance of the neurotransmitters in the synapse allow for a fast transfer of the impulse.) Another group of drugs, notably lithium and bupropion, work another way. These drugs inhibit the metabolism of these neurotransmitters.

There are many antidepressants out there to choose from. The overall efficacy is very similar for all of them. Most of the time physicians try one; if it doesn't work, they try another one. Drug companies who manufacture these drugs spend mass amounts of money promoting them. Other considerations as to *why* and *how* these drugs are prescribed are: (1) the adverse effect profile, (2) the type of presenting depression, and (3) any physical problems which a patient may have which would make the physician leery of prescribing an antidepressant.

The antidepressants available on the market are amitriptyline (Elavil), imipramine (Tofranil), nortriptyline (Pamalor), desipramine (Norpramine), doxepin (Sinequam), amoxipine (Ascendin), fluoxitine (Prozac), trazodone (Deseryl), and bupropion (Wellbutrin). Prozac is a selective re-uptake blocker that does not allow serotonin to "get back on the train." It also seems to work by creating a desensitization of the auto-receptors that inhibit the release of serotonin. The neurochemistry is quite complicated, and it's very likely that much more research needs to be conducted as to how and why all of this works.

Side effects are a major concern in prescribing antidepressants. The major side effects fall into four categories: (1) anticholinergic, (2) sedation, (3) orthostatic hypotension, and (4) cardiotoxicity. Often antidepressants are prescribed *because* of the side effects. For instance, sleep may be a big problem. Elavil or Deseryl has a proclivity toward sedation, so one of them is used. Drowsiness has been reported with nearly all antidepressants. Prozac and Wellbutrin, on the other hand, may cause insomnia or agitation. Anticholinergic side effects are primarily dry mouth, constipation, and blurred vision. Orthostatic hypotension takes place when you rise to an upright position and the blood pressure drops precipitously. Cardiotoxicity may become a problem, too. The cyclic antidepressants (amitriptyline, doxepin, and imipramine) may cause heart block, and they also have been known to cause seizures.

Newer preparations, like Prozac and Wellbutrin, have less side effects but they may "hop up" the PWCP, causing sleeplessness and agitation. Prozac may lead to weight loss, but usually it's not great. Sexual dysfunction may happen, but it usually resolves with time. Weight gain can be avoided by a controlled diet. Pain control is possible with much lower doses than those recommended to counteract depression.

Depression can result from internal biochemical abnormalities (endogenous depression). Situational dynamics can also cause depression. PWCPs definitely have reason to claim the situational dynamics which result in depression. On the other hand, studies of depressed patients have demonstrated that they definitely have a lot of complaints about pain. When the pain is secondary to depression, it's usually a headache, low back, dental, precordial (heart), or low abdomen complaint. Depression certainly presents a clinical challenge.

When true endogenous depression is present, antidepressants are definitely in order for the PWCP. Most physicians, particularly psychiatrists, are quick to prescribe them when the issue comes up. Depression is treatable by antidepressants and if there is any question, the patient with chronic pain will end up on antidepressants. Most antidepressants are expensive and require monitoring, which means lab work or office visits (usually both).

Antidepressants should be prescribed carefully and only with reserved judgment. A rule of thumb is that if a person who has chronic benign intractable pain can work a good Twelve Step path, such as the Chronic Pain Anonymous program advocated in Book II, and after a year or so thinks he or she is still depressed, looking into appropriate antidepressant therapy may be in order. At times these medications are highly recommended. For some, antidepressants are a godsend.

## The Bottom Line

The main problem in getting PWCPs off drugs is that most are psychologically locked into the notion that the "pills" or other drugs are their link to sanity and salvation. Those "awful addicts" get addicted of their own free will; *they,* on the other hand, are very different. Many people with chronic pain are totally convinced they cannot live without narcotics and other mind-altering substances. They can't conceive of a life without drugs to alleviate the pain. The mere thought of getting off drugs throws them into a panic, and it's most difficult to change a person of this mind-set. They don't think of themselves as "drug addicts," because drug addicts are "those people" on street corners and dark back alleys shooting up for pleasure.

Withdrawal from drugs is the same for anyone hooked on them, and all addicts hurt badly when they try to quit. They hurt until they get more of their drug. PWCPs hurt more when withdrawing, but once they get through it they are usually amazed to find it isn't all that bad. Some actually suffer much less as time progresses. The real plus is that, once they're drug free, they're John Doe or Mary Doe, not John or Mary plus a drug. They find they are different people, and others notice it, too. They sleep better, eat better, exercise more, help others, and so on. Without the drug dependency, PWCPs can start to work on healthy pain management. They launch a new life, a life with self-respect, fun, and a future. It may not be pain-free, but it's a lot better than what they had.

# The Importance
# of Exercise

▲    Probably the cornerstone in the management of chronic benign intractable pain is exercise, and that is not ecstatic news for anyone suffering from chronic pain. It's difficult to get people to exercise when they are feeling *well,* and PWCPs don't feel well most of the time. Motivation becomes a prime factor for them.

You may think of exercise as some vigorous physical activity resulting in copious amounts of sweat. An exercise program for a person with chronic pain may be entirely different, however. Most treatment facilities employ exercise physiologists who structure individual programs to fit specific needs. Some PWCPs can barely move without screaming; others get their pain primarily with the movement of specific muscle groups. Just about anyone, however, can benefit by performing some exercise which puts at least some strain on the heart and lungs. Once exercise is effectively put in motion and continued regularly, it seems that the pain diminishes steadily. At first the price may seem stiff, but as time progresses, it's well worth it.

It's no secret that PWCPs, as a rule, are in pathetic physical condition. Pain restricts physical exercise.

Poor muscle tone results, and that complicates the picture. The less activity performed, the more you feel like doing absolutely nothing. Weight lifters look great when they are routinely lifting; when they stop their exercise regimen, they become ordinary looking in a hurry. Muscles atrophy, and unless exercise is part of your life, your musculo-skeletal system will continue to go downhill. Public Enemy No. 1 in this case is pain.

It's a great thing for PWCPs to be involved in a pain management unit because most employ men and women who can think of fifteen different ways to strengthen musculature with a minimum of discomfort. They are also well-versed in using what's available for exercise. They can teach someone how to get a vigorous workout even while in a wheelchair, and it's hard for the PWCP to out-fox them. They're used to excuses and are also used to witnessing the difference exercise makes in turning a person's life around. If weight-bearing joints ache, they use the swimming pool. If the legs are gone, they help develop the upper body. If a patient can walk, they get them into a walking program. If they can jog, they push running. After the initial shock wears off, most patients with chronic benign intractable pain begin to see the value of specialized exercise programs. With exercise they are able to do twice as much for themselves. They sometimes surprise themselves by encouraging others to exercise. Again, the most difficult thing is just getting the PWCP motivated to do it. Encouragement is needed every step of the way.

## Why Exercise?

It's important to explain some basic physiology to understand why exercise works for the PWCP. Exercise is not just a good idea; it's an absolute necessity where chronic pain is involved. Here's the chain of events. When a person exercises, blood is moved along by a pump. The pump is the heart. When little demand is made on the heart, the pump becomes weak. Exercise strengthens the heart. When brought along intelligently, the stronger heart promotes a better blood supply throughout the body. Muscles require more blood when put under strain. The heart and the vessels have to be more efficient in making that blood available. Exercise, by improving blood supply, promotes tissue healing.

The nerves in your body don't exist in a vacuum. They need nutrients and must be kept alive. Blood supply plays a major part in making all of this happen. *Neuritis,* by definition, means inflammation of the nerve. *Neuropathy* means diseased nerves. Both of these conditions are facts of life for the PWCP, but exercise helps. Creating a better blood supply to the nerves helps heal pathology. If you get just 10% improvement from an exercise program, it's 10% that wasn't there before you started!

The heart is one big, important muscle, and it doesn't run on air. It has to be kept alive with a strong blood supply. When the heart pumps, it forces fresh blood into its own musculature. If the heart does not have enough blood feeding itself, *ischemia* results. Chest pain begins to radiate into the neck and left arm. When vessels carrying blood to the cardiac muscle become plugged, a "coronary" results. Unless other vessels can pick up the slack to the area, the heart muscle atrophies and if severe enough, it leads to a quick demise. Exercise opens new vessels around the deprived area. Smaller vessels feeding the injured tissue become larger due to demand, and whole new routes of blood supply are forced into use. Through exercise some men and women end up with a better blood supply than ever, even after sustaining a major coronary. The key factor in cardiac rehabilitation these days is exercise.

Few people today are not cognizant of cholesterol. High density lipoproteins (HDL) are good cholesterol. Low density lipoproteins are "bad." Cholesterol is one of several factors involved in the development of heart disease—it plugs up the arteries. Exercise (and a good, healthy diet) raises the level of good cholesterol (HDL) and lowers bad cholesterol levels in the blood, two wonderful side effects. Cardiologists are also very big on the use of exercise to raise the HDL and prevent arteriosclerosis.

When the brain is deprived of blood supply, tissue dies. Brain cells are lost forever—we do *not* grow new cells. When a sufficient amount of cells are robbed of blood, a "stroke" results. But when exercise is being performed, blood is pumped at an accelerated rate to the brain. Exercise promotes a healthy vasculature supplying blood to the brain and with it, hopefully, the nutrients supplied by a good diet. In promoting a better blood supply, it prevents strokes. PWCPs need a good blood supply to their brains. Lack of exercise leads to a sluggish blood supply, but a good exercise program helps the PWCP stay alert and bright.

Exercise helps you sleep well. It stimulates your appetite. It puts a spring in your step. It can make or break a "comeback" for a person in chronic pain. It also fits beautifully into a Twelve Step program.

The Twelve Step approach is a "do-it-yourself" process that this book will describe at greater length in later chapters. But suffice it to say here that responsibility for personal health falls to the person with the problem in Twelve Step groups. The responsibility in chronic pain used to be with someone else, something else. It was up to the surgeon, the physical therapist, the nurse, the psychiatrist, the pills—anything or anyone but the PWCP. People who go the Twelve Step route soon start to feel pretty good about themselves, and they should. Exercise is something positive PWCPs can do for themselves. Physical therapists can provide passive exercise, but even that requires some cooperation. Active exercise comes from within and is part of the "winning," take-charge attitude integral to the Twelve Step approach. Exercise plays a big part in this process.

## Your Aching Back

The low back is a particular source of agony and, unfortunately, a favorite target for chronic benign intractable pain. Back injuries account for one-third of all Worker's Compensation benefits. It's also a place where exercise can be of great benefit, particularly with a "failed back," those cases where patients become worse post-surgery. When the medical staff runs out of tricks, back exercises done with precision and fortitude have often produced remarkable benefits. Religiously performed, specific exercises have brought many a PWCP back to the point where life was worth living once more.

The primary aim of exercise in the low back is stabilization. The same is true of the neck. Strong muscles and ligaments go a long way towards making that happen. Abdominal muscles, back exterior muscles, and the iliopsoas muscles (the deep, thick internal muscles in the buttocks) have to be strengthened and kept in shape. Most people do their prescribed exercises for a few weeks or months, then forget about them. When musculature becomes weakened, though, the vertebra begin to move around. This causes stretching and pressure on the emerging nerves and pain flares again. Once acute low back pain leaves, a specific exercise program frequently can stave off future pain, but the program must be continuous. Exercise should never be stopped.

## Wonderful Water

One of the most beneficial ways for PWCPs to exercise is in water. Water buoys the body. It takes the strain off body parts. It throws the back into neutral. It takes weight off the knees. It turns out to be terrific for the cardiovascular system, too, since water offers resistance. Walking in the water for twenty minutes has benefits equivalent to two hours of walking on land.

Your heart rate should always be monitored to make sure your water exercise program is not too much, however. Following aerobic principles helps you not overdo it. Aerobic principles are really quite simple. Start with 220 and subtract your age. Take 70 to 80% of the result and you have your Training Heart Rate (THR). For instance, if your age is 40, subtract 40 from 220, which gives you 180. Eighty percent (80%) of 180 is 144; 70% is 126. That's your THR range. The THR should be maintained for twelve minutes in order to call any exercise "aerobic." Those are the approximate rules. Some exercise physiologists suggest shooting for 60% at first and exercising for about twenty minutes or so, gradually working up in subsequent sessions to 70% and 80%. The rule of thumb is to start slowly, but stick with it.

Working out aerobically three times per week maintains efficiency; less than three times a week, the efficiency is lost; more than three, efficiency is picked up. The heart rate is, of course, the pulse, and it helps to become proficient at taking your pulse. All it takes is a sweep hand on a watch. Count your pulse for ten seconds and multiply by 6, fifteen seconds and multiply by 4, thirty seconds and multiply by 2, or if you have the time, count for sixty seconds. Practice makes perfect.

Walking in water is wonderful exercise. Just about anyone can do it. Swimming is obviously better, but most people can't do it for twenty minutes. Swimming and jogging are probably the best exercises, but not many PWCPs can handle either. The pulse or heart rate is usually not an issue with either of these heavy exercises since the pulse almost always exceeds the Training Heart Rate. Walking in the water at their Training Heart Rate for twelve minutes is generally acceptable for most people with chronic benign intractable pain because of the buoyancy factor. It has provided substantial benefit for millions to the point of giving them a new lease on life. The joints become more mobile, the heart and lungs get their workout, and it gets the PWCP out of the house. It's not perfect, but almost.

Just don't try to walk *on* the water; only physicians can do that.

# The Mind's Role
# in Pain-Relief

▲   The mind plays a large part in the management of chronic benign intractable pain. Again, as it was with exercise, this is not the best news in the world for those people trying to live with chronic pain. PWCPs experience a great deal of mental anguish, so the "mental mastery" of pain sounds problematic.

In essence, telling someone they can use their mind to alleviate pain is not at all like letting them know "it's all in your head!" "All in your head" is a sad misconception. The pain experienced by a PWCP is frighteningly real. Physicians tell patients they can't find the *reason* they experience the pain. What they're saying is that they can't put a finger on the nociceptive input. It doesn't mean that the pain is imaginary. Pain specialists, algologists, firmly believe that once the pain is locked up in the central nervous system, people must learn to live with it— it doesn't have to mean the end of the world, however. There's much that can be done to ameliorate pain. The mind does have a tremendous influence over what can be done, and it isn't mystic or occult.

The prevalent thinking in the medical community

is that the mind is able to release special neurotransmitters, specifically endorphins, which drastically alter pain. This is not a "pie in the sky" theory. This is something concrete. Properly tooled, the brain can positively alter pain. It's an acquired skill, but it can help the PWCP manage the pain.

## Imagery

*Guided imagery* (sometimes called *clinical imagery*) is an important mental skill for managing pain. It has little to do with imagination. Imagination is aimless, scattered fantasy. Imagery is almost the opposite. Imagery is *focused*, requiring concerted concentration. Some of our most famous athletes have used guided imagery to set personal records. They learn through supervised practice to carefully perform their activities vividly in their minds before their particular events. They run through their events minutely, honing their skills, operating at 100%, perhaps several times, then they go out and break records. They visualize maximum performance, and then they physically accomplish their goals.

Clinical imagery is used for therapeutic purposes. It can be a therapeutic lifesaver. It has nothing to do with pills or invasive medical procedures. The mind is capable of producing powerful changes. Properly trained, patients are able to produce profound *physical* changes. Hypnotized patients can produce blisters on the skin by mere suggestion. The secret is in the ability to focus. You have probably witnessed remarkable feats performed by individuals in a hypnotic state. It's not by accident that the Indian fakir is able to sit on nails or walk on hot coals without injury. The secret is in the ability to focus, and the ability to harness this skill lies within each person. How does guided imagery work, and how can it be used to help manage pain?

When pain descends, most describe it in terms of burning, squeezing, piercing, numbness, pounding, crushing, etc. If pain represents a subjective image of "a ton of bricks landing on my chest," then that image is *countered* by picturing a hoist lifting the ton of bricks off the chest. This sounds simple enough, but guided imagery is an acquired skill and it requires much practice in order to be effective. All the senses must be utilized in the imaging. Exercises to heighten the sense of smell, touch, hearing, and sight have to be practiced constantly. The specific exercises in guided imagery involve size, color, depth, and motion. Successful results with the process require the ability to integrate the senses with special attention to detail. Some PWCPs respond better to the use of more objective images. For instance, if blood supply is the problem, they are able to vividly picture warm gloves, electrically charged, slipped over the hands with a temperature gauge they can regulate. They are trained to picture blood vessels being opened by a valve to increase supply. With the external heat of the gloves and the internal increase in blood flow, the limbs respond and pain leaves. Experts who specialize in guided imagery are available in most communities. They claim great success in working with people suffering from chronic pain.

## Biofeedback

*Biofeedback* is able to objectively measure bodily functions and immediately report the success or failure of imagery processes. Lights, bells, and displays tell the subject how much control is being exerted. PWCPs may feel they are moving heaven and earth during guided imagery, but unless the evidence is graphically displayed, it's back to work!

Results with imagery don't come easily, and biofeedback keeps people honest. It's easy to become discouraged if success is difficult to come by, but some PWCPs take to guided imagery quite fast. Either way, biofeedback provides objectivity. Once a person learns to mentally fly and the physical results are supported by biofeedback technology, they then can use the imagery by itself. When imagery doesn't seem to work effectively in the future, they go back to biofeedback for a refresher. Biofeedback eliminates much of the doubt that cynics are fond of using to destroy confidence. Biofeedback makes the PWCP walk his talk and work harder to achieve beneficial results.

## Modalities and the Twelve Steps

Anything that is reasonable and helps ameliorate pain fits right into a Twelve Step philosophy, and this book wholeheartedly advocates the formation of Chronic Pain Anonymous (CPA) groups based on the Twelve Steps of Alcoholics Anonymous. The one concession that is asked by any Twelve Step program is that the horse is kept in front of the cart. Chronic Pain Anonymous members can practice the philosophy and principles of AA and thereby keep their minds clear and free of turmoil. Exercise and guided imagery fit in admirably with the overall pain management program, but these and other modalities are not used to replace Twelve Step help. Specialists can sometimes take over a PWCP's pain program—the next thing you know, the Twelve Steps are on the back burner and deterioration begins.

Exercise helps immensely to strengthen the heart and lungs, loosen up the joints, firm up muscles, produce endorphins, increase appetite, promote sleep, and so on. Guided imagery brings the mind into play and the mind is a tremendously powerful tool that can be effectively applied to relieve pain. Guided imagery offers the PWCP an immediate tool that can be picked up and used on request. If the tool is not in good shape, however, or if the tool is rusted from neglect, it will be useless. The carpenter takes loving care of his tools, always practicing his or her craftsmanship. Guided imagery is one tool that can be used when pain becomes too much to handle. If practiced faithfully, the skill will be there to ensure performance. It isn't able to replace a Twelve Step program, however.

If the PWCP works the Twelve Steps, guided imagery and other modalities are more tools that can be counted on to work on the torment. When the mind is sharp, the heart pure, attitude tuned, conscience clear, and family discord replaced by peace— all part of Twelve Step activity—the PWCP can grab a tool like guided imagery or exercise and use it to help fight the war on pain. A good Twelve Step program will prepare the person suffering from chronic pain to latch on to modalities like exercise and guided imagery and use them effectively. A good Twelve Step program provides the overall framework for success in life. When this is understood and followed, the horse is out in front of the cart, where it belongs.

# Muscle Relaxation

▲   Pain creates tension, particularly muscle tension. And muscle tension hurts like fury. Have you ever witnessed a sprinter pulling up in a race and grabbing his or her legs? That's a graphic display of acute pain. Almost every athletic contest is punctuated by athletes rolling around on the floor or field from pulled muscles. Spasm is also painful. Being unable to move in bed because of muscle spasms in the low back is a good example of the agony muscle pain and spasm can cause. Feeling a muscle that has turned rock hard is likely to demand your attention, particularly when it feels like it's on fire.

When acute muscular pain is present, muscles stand out like boards. There's no need to feel the musculature—just look at it! Observe someone with acute back pain trying to get in and out of a chair. The grimace tells the story. In chronic benign intractable pain, most PWCPs have long forgotten what relaxed muscles are like. Any stress only adds to the muscle tension. It's like throwing wood on a fire.

## Focus on Relaxation

*Breathing techniques* are simple and effective methods of relieving muscle tension. Such techniques are among the oldest and most proven. A regular relaxation routine takes about twenty minutes and should be performed twice a day, if possible. It must be done in a quiet atmosphere and it should be uninterrupted. The exercise may be done sitting in a comfortable chair or lying down. Officially the process is called *controlled breathing.* The exercise is performed by taking easy, even deep breaths, and vocalizing one word when exhaling. The repeated word is one of choice. "Relax," "calm," or whatever you choose is repeated with each exhalation. Your eyes should be kept closed and your complete concentration is required. As soon as the exercise is completed, the resumption of your daily activities is suggested. Many PWCPs feel these twenty-minute periods twice a day are their best times of the day. After each session they feel refreshed.

*Progressive relaxation* techniques are similar to the breathing. They also take about twenty minutes to complete and require a peaceful, uninterrupted atmosphere. They can be done sitting in an erect posture or lying down. When you are relaxed as much as possible, focus your concentration on both feet. Curl your toes as tightly as possible for about ten seconds, then completely relax so that you can experience the blood supply and the relaxed musculature in your toes. Your complete attention is required. Next, tighten your legs as much as possible, hold for ten seconds, then relax. Focus your complete concentration on both legs. If done correctly, you will experience a sensation of heat caused by an increased blood supply to the area. When the exercise is properly performed, the muscles in your legs should be as limp as possible. Most people feel a heaviness which accompanies the increased vascular activity. The next area of focused concentration is the buttocks. Hold both buttocks as tight as you can for ten seconds, then completely relax. The progressive relaxation continues with the low back, followed by the upper back and neck, both arms, then abdominal and facial muscles. Most people experience a generally complete tension release and their pain is reduced. The term "progressive" here is obvious. You progressively move through each muscle group, and many claim their pain drains progressively. It can't be done occasionally to be effective, however. It has to be a daily routine, for the more a PWCP performs the exercises, the more proficient he or she becomes at achieving beneficial results.

*Autogenic training* is another technique that seems to provide consistent pain relief. Autogenic training originated in Germany, and it also takes about twenty minutes per session. It requires a quiet atmosphere and can be performed in a comfortable chair or in a reclining position. In this process you repeat certain phrases to yourself while focusing on a particular area of the body. For instance, you repeat the phrase "I can feel heaviness and warmth in my feet!" several times until your feet actually feel warm. When your feet *are* warm, you repeat the same technique for each contiguous body part. Like imagery, this takes concentration and vivid visualization.

Several relaxation techniques may be combined to provide desired levels of pain and tension relief. For instance, it makes sense to perform progressive relaxation and autogenic training on a warm, sunny beach. It would be great to perform them in a field of flowing wheat washed with sunlight. Through the force of imagery, the mind is able to transport you almost anywhere, anytime. It might help you to remember boring school days and how easy it was to fantasize. Any person of "average" abilities can use imagery to be transported to any beautiful, peaceful location. Also, the more you practice, the more skill you acquire. Proficiency and improved results come with practice.

## Relaxation 101

*Biofeedback* seems to be the technique of choice for relaxation training purposes. The reason is simple enough: it's an almost totally objective form of gauging progress. You can *think* your feet are warm or your hands are warm, but to objectively prove it is another matter. Biofeedback tells you immediately whether your techniques are working, and it gives you immediate reports.

When people are under stress, the hands and feet become cold. Initially, stress produces a surge of epinephrine. A flood of the drug epinephrine (also called adrenaline), causes immediate alertness and is one of the reasons our species has been able to survive. The heart speeds up, pupils dilate, and blood is forced to the vital organs. Epinephrine constricts blood vessels in the periphery of the body, and when this occurs, the limbs lose temperature. This is how stress physically causes a drop in temperature in the hands and feet and also causes the muscles to tighten. Very often you may subjectively feel "relaxed" when in fact little or no biological change takes place. PWCPs may think they are doing a great job performing progressive muscle exercises and autogenics, but they never really know with certainty without the benefit of feedback. Again, biofeedback provides that information instantaneously. With a better blood supply, pain should be alleviated. If there is no relief, then the relaxation exercise is not being done properly. Biofeedback visually demonstrates with objectively measured readings of the pulse, blood pressure, and muscle tension that the mind is causing *biological* changes to take place.

Most biofeedback training sessions last about an hour, and it takes several sessions for people to "catch on." Some are wonderful at it; others must work diligently in order to produce similar results. Some try too hard, but relaxation techniques are not meant to be forced. Obsessive-compulsive types often think they can *make* anything happen, but it simply doesn't work that way. The key to muscle relaxation is to *allow* it to happen. Tension doesn't abandon the musculature without training, and these techniques must be carefully learned and coached by a specialist who knows how to get the best results. One or preferably two sessions a week are routine in most chronic pain management units.

## Being Realistic

Biofeedback is specific for muscle tension. Stress, of course, causes tension. Biofeedback is a terrific tool, but it doesn't hold all the answers. If your pain is due to a biological cause like cancer or nerve damage, biofeedback will do little to relieve the pain. Arthritis pain will not "go away" by using biofeedback and these techniques. It's for muscle tension only. The use of biofeedback *reduces* pain, and anything that reduces pain should be looked upon as gold where chronic pain is involved. If it reduces pain 25 to 50%, it should be approached like an Olympic trial. All relaxation techniques should be viewed as a golden opportunity to turn your life around. The responsibility for pain management is always with the PWCP. Another person can't perform progressive relaxation, autogenics, biofeedback, or other techniques for you. If you are suffering from chronic benign intractable pain, you can't expect a miraculous "cure" either. Your gains with any technique may be small but at least they're gains. If you have chronic pain, then you have become used to setbacks. Your victories are rare. Success comes only through hard, tenacious work. If an easy answer were available, your pain would be long gone.

Using these techniques can be the beginning of a string of small victories that turn into big gains, however. Hits eventually do produce runs. Relaxation, autogenics, and biofeedback are not the "Holy Grail" to take your pain away, but they are hard-earned, proven modalities that help *lessen* pain. It's human nature to look for the quick cure, and the typical PWCP has had every imaginable fling at a "cure" with little or no luck. The results of trying have invariably led to more, not less pain. The techniques covered in this chapter offer a substantial glimmer of hope. Done properly, they may afford much more than just a glimmer.

One of the most positive aspects of these muscle relaxation techniques is that PWCPs do them. *They* earn a place in the winner's circle for a change. They get an opportunity to mount the podium and listen to the national anthem. A pill, a pill-pusher, a needle jockey, a surgeon, or an alternative health practitioner didn't do it for them—they did it. A person suffering from chronic pain needs this type of fresh experience. They need to look at the dials on a biofeedback machine and say, "By God, I'm doing it! I'm making this happen!" Imagery, relaxation techniques, and autogenics become something very real for the PWCP. Most have had their fill of hurt, hot air, and promises. Most like the idea of helping themselves and taking back some responsibility for their own health and wellness.

The last chapter noted the value of using positive pain management techniques with a Twelve Step program. A Twelve Step program says, "Take responsibility, get off the mark and do it, live again, be kind to yourself, make yourself the best person possible, live and let live, and take it one day at a time!" Muscle relaxation techniques fit into this philosophy very well, but the techniques and a Twelve Step program are only as effective as the person using them. The person suffering from chronic benign intractable pain must wrestle back control over his or her life. The proper use of these techniques, and their self-directed, responsibility-based focus, are certainly a big step towards regaining control, managing pain, and living a full life.

# Hypnotherapy

▲    All human beings have a conscious and an unconscious mind. The unconscious mind is vast and powerful. There are two components of the unconscious that function differently. The subconscious functions principally as a memory storehouse. The other part of the unconscious is called the superconscious (or super-ego) and deals with the spiritual aspects of self. *Hypnotherapy* gives you access to buried or suppressed information in your subconscious. It's one of the many modalities successfully used in the management of chronic pain.

There's not much question that pain causes tension, both physically and mentally. You know how you tighten your muscles when you're about to experience pain. When a blow is about to fall, the musculature becomes almost rigid. Pain causes tension, and you've learned well from personal experience. Stubbing your toe is painful. Heat burns your skin and causes pain. The mere thought of pain causes tension. Through hypnotherapy, you can learn how to relax the affected areas of your body which are physically causing you pain. With this relaxation comes an increase in blood circulation and a sense of overall lightness, warmth, and well-being. Any way you can learn to relax produces a pain-reducing effect. A PWCP needs to learn how to relax, and hypnotherapy has a proven record of doing just that. *Psychogenesis* is the development of physical disorders as the result of mental conflicts (rather than from organic causes). If there is a psychogenic component to your pain, hypnosis may prove therapeutic and effective, too.

Hypnosis has been around for some time. It was the sole anesthetic for major surgery during the first half of the nineteenth century. Ether and chloroform replaced it. With its "anesthetic effect," it's obvious that physiological pain resulting from acute trauma or disease can be relieved by hypnosis. Physicians, dentists, nurses, psychologists, and allied health professionals use it to relieve acute pain. Chronic pain is usually accompanied by fear, and it's rare when a PWCP doesn't have to deal with "emotional overlay." Fear of pain can be an overriding factor in the PWCP's daily life, and he or she is generally distraught from the ubiquitous pressures which accompany the chronic pain syndrome. If the tension and stress can be lifted through the use of hypnosis, the PWCP receives a great benefit. As stressed earlier in this book, *any* modality or method that affords the PWCP relief from pain should be utilized!

## Misconceptions

The efficacy of hypnosis depends on an individual's ability to respond to the treatment, and the results will vary. The hypnotic "formula" is based on the following: *Hypnosis equals Expectation; Expectation is catalyzed by Imagination; Imagination produces Belief; Belief, in turn, leads to Conviction and the desired therapeutic Results.* Many misconceptions about hypnosis have arisen in popular culture, primarily as a result of watching "Mandrake the Magician" types perform hypnotic acts in public. "Illusions" play a major part in their acts, but hypnotism is not of the occult, the world of magic, or the supernatural. It has a valid scientific basis and is really a manifestation of the human mind.

At one time it was erroneously thought that it was the skill of the hypnotist that determined the success or failure of the modality. The skill of the hypnotist is one factor, true, but the subject is usually the primary source of success or failure. In some cases, pain can be a PWCP's way of coping with emotional problems. If the PWCP uses pain as a tool to manipulate others, for instance, he or she will not benefit from hypnotherapy because they *need* pain in their lives. The subject of hypnosis will only achieve the results they honestly desire.

Many think that in hypnosis, the operator "dominates" the subject by his or her will. There is no domination or submission in hypnosis, however. The process works by allowing the subject to release and express their *own* intent or hidden abilities. Through the hypnosis process, subjects are unburdened of suppressed fears and doubts. The talent, inclinations, information, and will are with the subject; hypnosis merely allows the subject to function without restrictions.

One of the oldest and hard-to-kill fallacies about hypnosis is that someone can be hypnotized against their will. To be hypnotized, the subject must cooperate, and it takes full consent to cooperate. Many people may voice their consent, but their desire is absent. Some skeptics may become hypnotized, but underneath the bravado, they really do wish to experience the hypnotic state.

Probably a more serious and blatant falsity is the notion that a hypnotist has absolute control over a subject's mind and body. It's nonsense to think that a hypnotist can make a subject do or say anything contrary to their deep-rooted principles. Any suggestions that would arouse sincere moral indignation or repugnance immediately triggers a break in the trance, either by the subject resuming a "waking" state or lapsing into sleep. Hypnosis doesn't render you helpless. On the contrary, it's a vehicle to release and intensify your personal powers and abilities.

Some people harbor the notion that weak-willed, unintelligent people make the best subjects for hypnosis. There is nothing, however to do with willpower in this process; success with hypnosis depends heavily on the imagination. By far, the best subjects are strong-willed, intelligent, and creative. 90 to 95% of all adults can be hypnotized to some degree, not just a small segment of the population. The insane, infants too young to understand, and those who are intoxicated can't be hypnotized.

## Hypnosis How-To's

For PWCPs, it's advisable to undergo hypnosis only through someone who is a certified "hypno-anesthesia therapist." The certification process demonstrates that the hypnotist has been trained in the technique of pain management therapy. Specific contraindications for hypnotherapy are based on the therapist's training, skill, experience, and clinical objectives. The PWCP should become involved in the hypnotherapy process only after a medical referral has been made. For example, acute back pain may be simply due to muscle strain or sprain, or it may also indicate a herniated disc. Hypnosis, if applied *prior* to medical examinations, might mask the pain symptoms and leave the underlying cause for the pain untreated. In the case of chronic pain, however, this scenario is less likely. PWCPs have usually exhausted all medical avenues and have consulted innumerable physicians prior to seeking help through hypnotherapy.

When you first consult with a hypnotherapist, the initial meeting is used to establish rapport, determine therapeutic goals and objectives, and arrive at appropriate suggestions and preferred methods for inducing hypnosis. Hypnotic techniques will vary from person to person, so it will be important to determine precisely what might work for you. The initial interview is also an opportunity to answer questions and explain what happens when hypnosis is used. Oftentimes, simple suggestibility tests are tried out.

Many think that a hypnotist merely lulls a subject off to sleep. This would be accomplished by soothing words or soft music. This, however, is not the case. The state of hypnosis represents a condition whereby your *conscious* mind is completely relaxed and rested, without being put to sleep. You should be comfortable during the induction of hypnosis. There should be no weight or pressure on body areas which might impede circulation. With more permissive (versus authoritarian) techniques, a sound of quiet confidence will instill a desire in you for complete relaxation. Suggestions from the hypnotist must stimulate your imagination in order to produce a state of hypnosis.

When you achieve a relaxed state, therapeutic suggestions should be given to you in a manner that enables you to expect a desired outcome and enable you to use your imagination to produce the desired results. Therapeutic suggestions should begin with simple statements that are based on the positive results from the suggestibility tests given to you in your initial interview. Positive results from these tests will enhance your belief and conviction, will stimulate your imagination, and foster the belief and conviction that future suggestions will be accepted by your subconscious, producing the desired therapeutic results.

## Techniques

There are many specific techniques within hypnotherapy which seem to be beneficial for subjects. *Progressive relaxation,* outlined earlier, can be easily modified under hypnosis to produce a much greater depth of relaxation. As a whole, this technique will help you increase concentration and redirect your attention to health and wellness. Progressive relaxation can either be used under an "authoritarian" or a "permissive" approach with colorful imagery to enhance your relaxation, release stress, and lessen muscle tension.

Psychogenic (non-organic) pain may be managed with *imagery* that enables you to dissolve and dismiss pain. There is a type of imagery known as "Pain or Anxiety as the Object," and it's basically a technique where you imagine placing the pain outside of your body. Through imagery and hypnosis, you would give the source of your discomfort size, shape, and color. You would then practice increasing or decreasing the intensity of the color and size of the "object," thereby managing your externalized pain problem.

In *dissociation,* the subject receives some degree of relief from pain by allowing the PWCP to separate their body from their consciousness. This technique suggests to the PWCP that a certain body part is being perceived by the subconscious mind to be in another place or position than the body part is thought to be by the conscious mind. This empowers the PWCP to control or manage his or her "perception" of the pain and provides the powerful message that "you are not the pain."

*Disorientation* is a technique that can guide the PWCP to another place and time. When you leave a place or time of anticipated pain or discomfort, your subconscious mind perceives the pain stimuli as being only pressure. This technique is a great choice for elevating the PWCP's pain threshold.

*Glove anesthesia* is a hypnotic technique that allows the PWCP to anesthetize a portion of their body by touching that portion with their hand. The hand has already been made to feel numb through visualization and imagery, and that numbness is transferred from the hand to the area of discomfort.

With *safe place imagery,* the hypnotist helps the subject to facilitate disorientation and hypnotic analgesia (an insensibility to pain while still conscious). Hypnotic suggestions are given to the PWCP that they are in another place and time. That "safe place" that they are experiencing is free of any discomfort or unpleasant sensation.

*Self-hypnosis* is a technique that can be easily learned and used to relieve chronic pain. Many different methods are used to teach the techniques involved. Through self-hypnosis, you can reinforce therapeutic suggestions at home or at work. You must practice it daily in order to achieve results, but it's very worthwhile. This is one of the most important elements of the hypnotic procedures found in any good pain management therapy program.

# Group Therapy

▲   Group therapy is a staple in most pain treatment or general medical facilities. It's there for a reason: group therapy is effective. It's tough for a PWCP to "hide out" in group therapy, and people with chronic pain tend to do a lot of hiding out. Pain drives people to retreat inside themselves. Even extroverts become subdued when acute or chronic pain visits. With chronic pain, the unwelcome visitor stays and destroys the host unless steps are taken to gain control. Group therapy helps the PWCP gain that control. One-to-one therapy is generally preferred by most patients, but less beneficial work gets done. One-to-one sometimes turns into a test of wits or a match of minds. Groups, by contrast, tend to be more open and honest. People who like to hide out don't usually like group therapy—but it's good for them.

The great thing about this therapy is that it affords the PWCP an opportunity to vent anything negative ("dump the garbage") in the presence of peers. It's tough to con a con in a group setting. Personal dishonesty is quickly picked up on and confronted. Many self-styled "intellectuals" don't care for this type of therapy. They can dazzle a therapist one-to-one, but a group generally challenges them in a hurry. Introverts have a hard time introverting. Groups tend to drag introverts from their shells. Once out, some introverts like the climate and it's hard to keep them from talking. Most introverts are inclined to think a great deal, but they don't express their feelings well. With some, the release of thoughts, feelings, convictions, humor, anger, disappointments, frustrations, rebelliousness, and bitterness is somewhat akin to opening up the flood gates, and that great release is very therapeutic.

## Session Dynamics

Group therapy is a chance to "let it all hang out." With chronic pain, the PWCP's feelings are generally locked up. "Frozen feelings" is an apt term applicable to most, and they are filled with hurt. Some PWCPs dare anyone to try to draw them out. In group, hostility can gradually turn into amicability once risks are taken. Unfortunately, some PWCPs hang back for weeks without participating. By the time they decide to open up, opportunity has passed them by and group treatment has almost come to a close. Weeks are often wasted where much work could have been accomplished.

It soon becomes apparent in group therapy that everyone has something unique to offer. Wisdom is not always the exclusive property of the more educated members of the group. So often, the less voluble make the most sense. Introverted men and women do much listening, and they tend to learn more. PWCPs are just everyday people who happen to be saddled with chronic pain. They are no different, no smarter, or no less intelligent than other people. They somehow fell into the pit of chronic pain where God doesn't seem to differentiate between introverts and extroverts. People from all walks of life, intellectual pursuits, financial status, races, and creeds fall into disease and addictions with regularity. Groups tend to end up with a potpourri of interesting men and women who get to share their learnings and wisdom—and they tell it as it is. Honesty is most important.

In chronic pain management and chemical dependency programs, group therapy is usually directed by a therapist. Most of them are well educated and have had a wealth of experience. Their job is to see that everyone in the group gets as much out of each session as possible. Sometimes therapists come off as calloused, but it's their job to keep people on track. They're not supposed to be cheerleaders. They're in the therapy setting to see that the group does not exceed boundaries and cause unnecessary hurt. Therapists are trained to recognize when individuals have been taken down the road too far. For the most part, they're dedicated, sharp professionals who earn their money ten times over. They work long hours and they also get worn out fast. Many can take the pace of therapy sessions for only so long.

In past chapters there has been an analogy drawn between the PWCP and the addict. Likewise, a program on the order of Alcoholics Anonymous can also benefit the person suffering from chronic pain. In a sense AA *is* group therapy. Members from all strata of society tell their stories, help each other out, and carry their self-honesty back into their daily lives. There are no professional leaders in AA, unlike in group therapy, but AA seems to get along without them. AA and other Twelve Step program adherents follow the principles, philosophy and traditions of AA, and they get their group work done through them. The bonus with AA is that the process costs nothing but personal time and effort.

A version of AA that would function solely for PWCPs, Chronic Pain Anonymous (CPA), would operate in classic AA fashion. People with chronic pain would show up at meetings and talk about how pain affects their lives, how they are learning to cope with it, and what pain management tools work for them. PWCPs would freely admit that pain has made their lives unmanageable and they are powerless over their pain, just like an alcoholic is powerless with booze.

There are meetings in AA where Steps are the prime subject. Every meeting means a new Step, and the group simply takes one Step apart and works it over. By the end of the meeting, everyone comes away with new insight. "Step" meetings are commonplace in every community. CPA, of course, would have to apply the principles and philosophy of the Twelve Steps to chronic benign intractable pain. This process will require people who have "been there." When PWCPs dissect a Step, it will take on a different, more pain-specific aura.

Years ago it seemed that "pure" alcoholism or "pure" heroin or cocaine addiction was the rule. That's not so today. Most addicts today are into multiple drugs. Many smoke crack, use pot regularly, are heavy drinkers, and 80% are addicted to cigarettes. PWCPs can readily apply the principles and philosophy of AA to their chronic pain condition and thereby change their lives. Since most are into multiple drugs, too, there is no reason why they cannot participate in other Anonymous meetings, radiating out from their core of support at CPA. Many PWCPs can go from a treatment center, transfer to an outpatient status, then go on to CPA for a lifetime involvement. Any route will do as long as the PWCP desires to live a whole life. The more seasoned PWCP may be a great source of help to those who could not afford the treatment route. Those lucky members may have picked up newer techniques that have benefited them and, in turn, they can willingly share their experience in a CPA setting. Throwing patients with the common background of chronic pain together for an hour or so will definitely benefit some individuals, and when the principles and philosophy of a Twelve Step program provide the structure, nothing but good can surface.

Where chronic pain is concerned, a patient's aftercare has a history of falling apart post-treatment. With CPA, things would not necessarily fall apart. The PWCP's gains would be stabilized and capitalized upon in the group setting. Families would also get support through their own CPA-related group (after all, AA has Alanon and Alateen, and NA has Naranon). PWCPs should attend many CPA meetings—the more, the better. For starters, "90 in 90" (ninety meetings in ninety days) should be the minimum. If no CPA meeting is available in the PWCP's community, an AA or NA meeting will suffice. Every CPA member should be able to say with pride that "90-90" was his or her first victory. Every sponsor should obligate his or her charge to reach the 90-90 goal. Such advice is usually met with much wailing and gnashing of teeth, but it does pay off. Keep in mind the traditional AA "$100 principle." If someone stood outside the door passing out $100 bills to members as they entered, and the door was closed at the appointed hour, two things would happen. One, members would probably go to three meetings per day. Two, they would be fifteen minutes early to meetings. Arnold Schwarzenegger wouldn't be able to hold out the crowd! If PWCPs attended

Twelve Step meetings as if the $100 principle applied, their lives would improve. Group therapy works, and group experiences within the AA tradition can become a valuable key to the success of their lifelong aftercare program.

# Don't Forget the Families!

▲    One of the most important components of a strong treatment program is the Family Program. It's most distressing to pull a person out of his everyday environment, educate him, treat his chronic pain, and then place him back in the same unchanged home atmosphere and expect a favorable outcome. It isn't fair to the patient and it isn't fair to his family.

"Families" encompass more than blood relatives. Significant others must be included. Actually anyone who lives with or is closely associated with PWCPs should be included in the treatment process. The addiction field learned long ago about the near-fatal wounds inflicted on those surrounding anyone dependent on drugs. Deep scars, bewilderment, anger, disgust, mental problems, codependency issues, physical maladies, and ignorance of drug issues, to name a few, are all conditions commonly found in the families of those addicted to drugs. These issues may be of much greater magnitude in the family of one suffering from chronic benign intractable pain.

One of the major problems encountered among family members is codependency. The wife, husband, daughter, son, sister, or brother may take on the responsibility of "fixing" the person with chronic pain. Not only is this impossible, it's wrong, and often as a result the codependent ends up in a worse lot than the one in chronic pain. What's even more detrimental is that codependency puts the PWCP in a position where change never takes place. As long as someone else "picks up the pieces," there's no reason to change.

Wives, husbands, and partners wait side by side in physicians' offices and emergency rooms. Quite often the partner is very caring, very comforting, and terribly concerned. He or she is also very agitated and worn out from running around for prescriptions, medical supplies, insurance forms, etc. For the most part, they suffer in silence, but they tend to be furious beneath the surface. The partner often becomes drained, wanting to help, wanting to see their partner, their son, their daughter, or their friend get well. But of course, with chronic pain, getting completely well usually doesn't happen. Family members become frustrated and angry. They sometimes can't help but show their true feelings now and then, and when that happens, "trench warfare" ensues. Most PWCPs get to be good counter-punchers and relationships are soon pushed to the limits. Resentments become a way of life. Even the martyrs sooner or later crumble and their resistance topples.

People with chronic benign intractable pain can learn to use their pain like a sword. Most do not, of course, but some become masterful manipulators. They can learn to rule the household, using pain as their whip. When confronted, a sharp PWCP can make the confronter feel lower than a snake's Adam's apple. Any PWCP worth his or her salt can make most people feel extremely guilty. The sad truth is that this control and dysfunction takes place so subtly that family members are in major trouble before they realize what's going on.

Most of the time, the family of a PWCP needs help in learning to cope. They need to learn, along with the patient, that changes have to be made. The disease of alcoholism and other drug addiction makes the addict sick, in so many ways, and their families also get sick. The same thing happens to the families of people with chronic pain. Some family member may become physically sick trying to cope with the PWCP. Hypertension, ulcers, colitis, headaches, coronaries, strokes, nervous disorders, anxiety, or depression may surface in the family members as they enter into their relationship with chronic pain. The partner of a PWCP often expires at a relatively early age and the PWCP survives. Some PWCPs are so tough, you can't proverbially kill them with an axe. The partner and close family members, however, die waiting on them.

## Help for Families

Family therapy is bound to play an integral part in the recovery program for any PWCP. Most of the best chronic pain management facilities and just about all the class chemical dependency units devote almost as much time to the families as to the PWCPs. Few care to take issue with the fact that everyone around the PWCP needs to be educated, vent their frustrations, and develop a game plan post-treatment which will best benefit all family members. A family's post-treatment plan must be reasonable and separate from the PWCP's. The family must be taught that they can't make the PWCP "well." The family's responsibilities must be separated from the PWCP's; the issues, for one, are completely different for the parties. The PWCP has his or her recovery and pain management program; the families have to look after their own mental health.

A comfortable meeting of the minds prior to the PWCP's medical discharge produces remarkable harmony when the PWCP returns to the family environment. Family involvement in the treatment process helps immensely. Family members become aware and vigilant of recidivism signs. They're prepared for the possible failures of the PWCP, and they learn that they must not shoulder the blame for these failures. Families become aware that they have their own problems and program to follow, helping the PWCP best by keeping themselves healthy. Hopefully, in a family therapy program all members will receive answers to their questions and be able to travel the same road with the PWCP—for a change.

TLC (tender loving care) is an important part of life. People would not be human if they didn't look for and appreciate earned strokes. TLC in chronic pain, however, can be overdone and even prove fatal. TLC plays an important part where acute pain is involved; with chronic pain it can lead to an "enabler" role that is suicide for the PWCP and his or her family. TLC must be used with discretion because it may reinforce pain and cause dependent conduct—a family member can unintentionally sabotage a great pain management program with too much TLC. Kindness is always the rule, and being reserved in chronic pain management may at times be interpreted as being stern and uncaring. No one likes to play "first sergeant," nonetheless, family members must learn to be both kind and firm. It's a way of relating to the PWCP that must be assumed before any progress can be made. PWCPs and their families need to be upfront with each other so they're able to blow the whistle when they catch each other falling back into their old negative behavior patterns. Alcoholism is truly a family disease, and so is chronic pain.

It's important for everyone to receive encouragement and just praise. Phony praise never works, but earned praise is good. A PWCP needs positive praise very, very badly because for one thing, they aren't used to it. Many people respond so well, they get carried away and overdo it, particularly with exercise. That may result in setbacks, not progress. Praise and encouragement must be dispensed judiciously to the PWCP with love and kindness, but only when it's deserved. Families need to let the PWCP know how much progress has been made and how they love and appreciate all their efforts, but the praise has to be genuine. People with chronic pain are sensitive, and hollow praise will sound phony to them. Praise only for performing good works; with chronic pain, it's necessary to reinforce only the positive. Positive praise often results in a more sincere effort by the PWCP.

One piece of deleterious conduct that never seems to sit very well in chronic pain treatment is "nagging." The quickest way to get an alcoholic back into the bottle is by perfecting this practice. Nagging a PWCP may produce a great deal more harm than good. *Reminding* someone of their responsibilities is occasionally all right; becoming the other person's conscience is counterproductive. It's always difficult for caring people in the PWCP's family to let go.

"Fixing" is what all well-meaning parents and all controlling relatives would like to do. You can't "fix" a PWCP, however. Defeating chronic pain must come from within. No one else can do it for the other guy. It's very difficult to relinquish control. Wives kill with kindness, husbands kill with kindness, and parents kill with kindness when it's misdirected. "Controlling" people in the PWCP's family have their own needs and they must work them out on their own, not through manipulating the PWCP. Control needs to go back to the one with the chronic benign intractable pain.

*Loss of control* is a major characteristic of all addictions; it's a major characteristic of the chronic pain syndrome, too. The patient needs to take back command and responsibility. Some family members have an unhealthy need to stay in control and simply refuse to let go. They are hell-bent on fixing. Many family members who are the most flagrant violators are shocked and bewildered to realize that they are filling this negative role. It's just one more reason to involve the entire family in the treatment process. The sooner the family environment becomes healthier for everyone, the more whole and healing the entire pain management process will be. A good family program is vital for everyone concerned.

# Pain Centers and CD Units

▲ Chronic pain syndromes are characterized by a preoccupation with pain, loneliness, passivity, lack of insight, and an inability to take care of your own needs. How can a treatment or management program address all these issues at the same time? Traditionally the treatment for chronic pain was bed rest, physical therapy, pain medication, more surgery, or nerve blocks. The outcome for the most part was relatively dismal. Chronic pain management centers were developed to meet the challenge of providing more effective care. When one approach doesn't seem to work, people try something else. If that seems to work, then they try to perfect the model. The "pain center" evolved just such a *multidisciplinary* approach.

## Entering a Program

What type of patient meets the criteria for a chronic pain management unit? The criteria are generally (1) someone who has responded poorly to conventional therapy, and (2) a person whose pain has caused significant dysfunction in their home, social, and work life. A majority, 50 to 70%, of those who qualify for admission have low-back problems, with two to three surgeries under their belts. All varieties of pain are addressed in treatment: neuropathies, headaches, facial pain, causalgia, joint pain, neck and back pain—just about any chronic pain that disrupts and destroys everyday function.

If a medical workup is indicated, appropriate consultations and tests are done following a good medical history and physical. The pain management programs consist primarily of group therapy, physical therapy, guided imagery, breathing techniques, progressive relaxation, autogenics, biofeedback, mild analgesics (aspirin or acetaminophen), ice and heat, and other modalities. If there is a drug problem, the withdrawal procedure commences. The goals, of course, are to restore function to the PWCP's lifestyle, get the patient to a drug-free state, treat the underlying depression and insomnia (if present), and decrease future medical care costs.

## Breaking the Habit

There are many different ways to accomplish the difficult task of getting a PWCP off narcotics. Many healthcare professionals, based on their experiences in pain care, believe that as many as 50% of PWCPs are addicted to medication (minimally), but every case is a little different. Most patients readily agree that the narcotics they came into treatment with did not relieve their pain. They relate personal horror stories of being "half in the bag" a good part of the time, dysphoric, and generally getting more and more out of touch. In other words, they were "out of control." All agree that narcotics and other mind-altering agents did not provide an answer to their chronic benign intractable pain.

All pain treatment facilities use some "deceleration" method for these PWCPs. This simply means that the narcotic dose is tapered over a period of time until the patient is drug-free. Decreasing doses, however, are very difficult to manage for people in outpatient programs. One method of deceleration is to pack all the drugs in decreasing doses into the pills dispensed daily to the PWCP. Patients line up for the same amount of "medication" daily, but they get decreasing amounts and they are aware of it. They never know how much dosage they will be getting. Pharmacists prepare the pills, and they are the only people who really know the dosages. They get the original directions from physicians, and from then on it's merely a matter of pill preparation and dispensing. This deceleration technique works very well.

Another method is to switch to another narcotic, say methadone, and administer it in decreasing doses. A third way is to use the same drug that the patient is "hooked" on and delete doses on a schedule. It's a matter of preference of the medical director which regime seems to fit in best for the patient, staff, and overall program. All of the systems seem to be effective. Getting addicts off pills isn't the big problem; keeping them off, unfortunately, is a different story.

## The Pain Center Approach

Once in treatment, whether inpatient or outpatient, the daily schedules keep the PWCP busy in a pain center program. Group therapy, medical management, physical therapy, occupational therapy, acupuncture, biofeedback, relaxation techniques, TENS unit therapy—all of these are usually worked into the program at one time or another. Many of these modalities are one-to-one and therefore require tight supervision and scheduling. One-to-one therapy is expensive, so costs tend to be high in hospital settings. Insurance companies have forced most chronic pain management units to go strictly outpatient primarily because of expense, but some offer both in- and outpatient programs. Some patients start a program while they're hospitalized and revert to outpatient status after several weeks.

Facilities that specialize in chronic pain ordinarily do wonderful work, but they have a weakness. Unless the patient lives in the immediate vicinity, their therapy ends when their treatment ends. Even if the patient lives next door to the hospital, expense limits aftercare. For this reason much of the "rebuilding" is lost for the PWCP. Patients tend to leave the pain center with a new attitude, good physical conditioning, a good game plan for an upbeat future, much less pain, and a pill-free system. In a sense, they have a new lease on life. When the PWCP hits the door, the hospital personnel usually are pleased, the patient feels very good about the whole process, the family is more intact, but there's still a problem— pain treatment ends. Without a good solid support and aftercare system, something very important is missing in these programs. If the gains are not *held*, both the pain unit and the patient suffer. If the patient is not a success, neither is the facility, and everyone loses!

## The CD Program Approach

Drug and alcohol programs (also called chemical dependency or CD programs) abound in our society. True, due to insurance pressures, fewer and fewer CD facilities are surviving, but presently they're still plentiful. All drug and alcohol programs admit chronic pain patients. Based on daily case management loads, easily 10% of an ordinary census consists of patients inflicted with chronic benign intractable pain. Those PWCPs have decided they have had their fill of narcotics and other mind-altering agents on their own, or some crisis has precipitated their admission into the CD program. Overdosing is not unheard of where chronic pain is involved. It's much more common, however, to see people in such programs who realize that drugs are wiping them out. They get fed up with having to beg for prescriptions. They hate the expense of hospital and office visits. They tire of conning other people. They grow weary of trying to convince family and friends that their pain is real, not just "in their heads." They become confused from the "fruit salad" menu of pills they are prescribed. Also, most PWCPs seem to eventually wind up drinking. Most of all, they come into a CD program because they see themselves as being on a treadmill, getting nowhere. Their pain is just as bad as ever. They realize the answer doesn't lie in the bottle or a pill and they want out. Most PWCPs sooner or later understand that they are "hooked," and there must be a better way.

Strangely enough, some people with chronic pain are pleasantly surprised when the drugs are slowly removed from their systems. The withdrawal itself is never easy, but they do live through it. They don't sleep for a while (many can't sleep well for months), but it gets a bit better every day. Benzodiazepines, if used, are sorely missed and present a major problem, but PWCPs make it. You can't alter your brain chemistry for several years and not expect to pay a big price during withdrawal. For every bit of sedation, agitation is the price. It's also a lot to expect patients to all at once accept modalities like exercise, meditation, relaxation, cold and heat applications, aspirin and acetaminophen, walking in the water, prayer, working on the First Step, or reaching out to others. It all requires the dedication of a skilled team of professionals, and this is precisely why the withdrawal from drugs is difficult to manage as an outpatient.

Patients need constant support and assurance. Many PWCPs walk out of treatment. This is particularly true when benzodiazepines are involved, and it seems the older the patient, the tougher the withdrawal, particularly with tranquilizers.

The peculiar problem that patients with chronic pain have to deal with in a chemical dependency facility is the *other* patients who are not being treated for chronic pain. Since they indeed are all dependent on drugs, they are involved with exactly the same program structure. Most likely, a Twelve Step program is offered because it's the best treatment currently offered. If CD patients wholeheartedly embrace the recovery philosophy and sincerely follow its principles, they live. If they don't, they die all too soon. (It sounds dramatic but most of the time, it's absolutely true.) In CD treatment, all patients do a First Step, find a sponsor, do ninety meetings in ninety days after they're discharged, and they go on to live reasonably normal lives with one major difference. If they follow the principles and philosophy, they have more fun, more money, and they enjoy the love and respect of their peers and family. They also end up helping others. PWCPs are perfectly capable of traveling the same road, but most seem to bump into an insidious roadblock that scuttles their progress. The roadblock is that they're *different* from the other drug-dependent people going through the treatment process with them. When their peers leave treatment, they're drug-free and own an AA, CA, or NA road map to aftercare success. PWCPs leave with some of the pain they came in with, but no good support group. That is their dilemma. "OK, so I'm off my pills. What the hell am I going to do with my pain?" The great majority do not stay clean because of it.

## Better Aftercare for the PWCP

For PWCPs in a pain center program, it would seem a natural part of the treatment process, inpatient or outpatient, to introduce the principles and philosophy of AA. If a patient accepted the Twelve Step program approach, a solid, practical, essentially no-cost aftercare program would be in place permanently. The beauty of a special Chronic Pain Anonymous (CPA) program is that it would throw people together with the common thread of chronic pain. Along with the spirituality of the Twelve Step program, the practical techniques picked up in treatment, like exercise, imagery or relaxation methods, would be natural subjects of discussion. Therein lies the support badly needed by the PWCP. The Twelve Step principles have given strength and solace to individuals and their families for over fifty years. If an individual left treatment having completed the First Step, it would serve as a foothold into a different, hopeful, and satisfying life. It would be the PWCP's invitation into a life requiring socialization, taking responsibility, and eventually sharing with others.

The adding of CPA meetings to the curriculum in a chronic pain treatment program would not be difficult. CPA essentially runs itself. Any good, interested AA member could help set them up. The better chemical dependency programs have dozens of experts in their employ. Borrowing or hiring someone from this discipline would be simple enough. Patients would naturally need professional guidance working the Steps. Some patients advance to Steps Two and Three in treatment, but it's Step One that sets the stage. The typical chronic pain management personnel would probably not be equipped to work with PWCPs on the concept, but almost all organizations, regardless of what the business, harbor Twelve Step members in their midst. It only takes one person who works a good program, one who unabashedly admits that his or her program has made the difference between living and dying, to get a CPA group started.

If every chemical dependency unit operated several Chronic Pain Anonymous meetings while PWCPs were in treatment and offered multiple meetings in the community when they were discharged, they would have a built-in support system where PWCPs could feel comfortable. Other CPA members may or may not have been addicted to drugs, but all of them have chronic pain. All of them relate to the peculiar problems facing the daily struggle of getting on with their lives without faltering. At a typical AA, CA, or NA meeting, you are likely to run into a PWCP, but at a CPA meeting, there would be nothing but people suffering from chronic benign intractable pain. If the meetings are conducted with the same seriousness as other Anonymous groups, much work will take place and the members will leave with hope and encouragement. They will also be exposed to new ideas, different approaches to pain management, new faces, a dose of reality therapy, and a beautiful philosophy of life. The PWCP would be able to pick up practical suggestions and encouragement to follow through with pain-ameliorating modalities. There would be many benefits, and no monetary cost for this unique form of aftercare!

Rubbing elbows with peers and relating personal experiences and preferences are bound to happen, and where chronic pain is concerned, it's healthy.

What helps one person may help another. Relating a bad experience may save someone else a similar ordeal. People who have been lucky enough to go through treatment in a CD or chronic pain management unit need to share what works for them. However, the Sixth Tradition in the AA "Big Book" must be honored. The traditions of AA succinctly point out that no Anonymous group should "endorse, finance, or lend the AA (or CPA) name to any related facility or outside enterprise less problems of money, property, and prestige divert us from our primary purpose." A PWCP will go to meetings for strength and unity. Carrying banners and extolling personal causes from a specific unit or CD program can be disastrous. It would drive people away. AA is a program of attraction, and CPA is a program of attraction.

Anyone who has chronic benign intractable pain and wants help should be welcomed with open arms at any CPA meeting. If someone has been through a chronic pain management unit, it's likely he or she left with many useful and practical therapies for alleviating pain. Hopefully, this person was exposed to CPA and completed at least the First Step. If a PWCP has gone through a CD unit, he or she knows all about AA and has a good background. Their strength should be a Twelve Step program. Sharing good experiences from the disciplines of pain centers and CD programs will enrich the CPA experience. The melding of experiences will be synergistic. People who wander in with neither experience may have a more difficult time, but it shouldn't be a deterrent. Addicts have been wandering into AA for fifty years armed with nothing but a desire to quit, and they make it. The better prepared the PWCP is, the more likely the success in aftercare or CPA group work. It's likely that more people who haven't had either a pain center or CD program experience will go directly into CPA. All PWCPs have the desire to quit the destructive behavior that seems to be entangled with chronic pain. They desire to learn what they can do to live useful and meaningful lives. All have experienced frustration and failure trying to get rid of pain, and all will have much to contribute and benefit from in working a Twelve Step program.

# Victimization or Change

▲   Many PWCPs perceive themselves as victims. Some get the notion that God is punishing them for past transgressions. God is somehow getting even by giving them pain. Their sins are of such magnitude that chronic pain is a just sentence for a lousy life. The PWCP can often become a professional victim. To a certain extent, all of us at times become victimized. It's part of life, but when victimization becomes part of your character and lifestyle, trouble brews on the horizon. When a PWCP falls into the "victim's hole," it results in much trouble.

Victims don't do a whole lot. The word "victim" connotes a person or thing about to be sacrificed or killed. The head is on the guillotine, and the fight is long gone. A person who has fallen into the "victim's hole" would not want anything to do with a Twelve Step program or healing/wellness modalities. Victims are like cattle standing around waiting to be slaughtered. A well-balanced pain management program is more for people who resemble war prisoners trying to escape a terrible fate—they're willing to do just about anything to improve their lot.

It's not hard to see how a person who is suffering from chronic benign intractable pain can stumble into the "victim's hole." With chronic pain nothing goes well. When people hurt, they tend to share the hurt by lashing out, and people around them lash back. Very few ever understand what's going on. Family members get mightily angered at the poor guy with the pain. They can't understand why the pain doesn't leave, and they start thinking the PWCP is crazy. Friends, family, physicians, physical therapists, clergy, and fellow workers (if there is still a job) descend *en masse* on him or her, and it isn't long before the PWCP begins to feel like a punching bag. Gloom and doom ensue. If they're normal human beings, they become depressed, and who wouldn't? They need to find some way to climb out of the hole. Victims quit trying, however. They become truly powerless. Their lives become unmanageable.

The first of the Twelve Steps is designed to show a person with chronic pain just how woeful life has become (all Steps will be thoroughly covered later on in Book II). Performed honestly, the First Step helps many PWCPs realize just how powerless they have become. Most don't like what they see. Many recognize the victim's role they have assumed and they want out. They recognize a need for change, and start by placing one foot on the ladder, slowly climbing out of the hole. The first rung on the ladder may be the successful graduation from a chemical dependency treatment center or a stay in a chronic pain management unit. The first rung on the ladder may be right off the street into a Chronic Pain Anonymous meeting.

Taking charge of your life is a big step in the right direction. Most PWCPs have left responsibility in the hands of others. Surgeons, "needle freaks," psychiatrists, psychologists, and other professionals have run the show. Victims allow others to control their lives. They pursue more surgery and receive more misery. Victims generally do nothing but line up for the next boot to kick them even harder. Accepting responsibility is something very new for them, and moving the professionals into the background and taking charge of their own lives is quite a new experience.

Victims, as a rule, are absolutely angry. Even victims who seem to almost *enjoy* their pain tend to be mad as hell. Anger and hostility seem to go with the territory, and a diehard victim is content to stay in the hole with the anger and watch the world go by. For many PWCP victims, their favorite game is "kick me." The First Step dramatically demonstrates to most that unless the person with chronic pain terminates the "kick me," "poor me" attitude, the victim role will never change. To someone looking in, the problem seems obvious and the need to change is even more obvious. To many PWCPs, however, the hole seems too deep and the climb out too steep. Pain paralyzes them. Chronic pain equals chronic torture, and the situation can easily be interpreted as completely and utterly hopeless. Friends, family, and professionals can easily stand on the sidelines and cheer, but it's far more difficult for the PWCP.

## A Difficult Choice

There are only two options for the PWCP's life. One choice is to continue down the same road of past victimization. It's unfair to be too critical of those who make this choice. It's always easy to see clearly how futile and defeating it is to continue down the same destructive path when the problem is not ours. When an intervention for substance abuse fails, many heavy hearts result. When the motivation is love for the person with chronic pain, a formal intervention may take place (and occasionally fail) but there should be no heavy hearts. Family and friends get together and give it their best shot. It means they tried to get the PWCP to see that help is needed.

If dramatic change doesn't take place, then the devastation, so common to all addicts and chronic pain patients, will continue. The choice is entirely theirs. At least those who have taken part in the intervention process have had the satisfaction of knowing they did all they could. Wringing the hands helps very little. When the choice is made that the PWCP is unwilling to make definite change, it should be a clear message that he or she prefers the old dysfunctional lifestyle. If chronic pain presents no problems, why change? If family and friends, through an intervention, fail to convince the person suffering from chronic benign intractable pain that all is *not* well on the home front, job and social life, at least they come away with the satisfaction of having given it their best.

Studies have shown that many skid row residents want it no other way. They like the lifestyle. The average man or woman finds that information unbelievable, but it's true. Some addictionologists feel that heroin addiction is as much an addiction to the lifestyle as it is to heroin. Alcoholics are frequently addicted to the lifestyle. Change is hard in each of these cases. Spending several hours in a bar every night for twenty years, and suddenly stopping it overnight is a tall order. People miss the camaraderie, the talk, banter, companionship, friends, smoke, and "fun," as they see it. They're addicted to the lifestyle, and some refuse to give it up. They lose their family, friends, and job, they spend time in and out of jail, they end up penniless, but that's what they prefer. And so be it—it's their choice.

Some PWCPs prefer their lifestyle. They don't mind being waited upon. Not having a job isn't all bad. You can sleep in every morning. As long as the benefits hold up, there's some money coming in. Family members can be kept in line by using the pain. The lawyers are pleased to share in the Worker's Compensation. Physicians sometimes become concerned because they see no progress in their patients, and they eventually might worry about the State Board of Licensure investigating their narcotic prescription patterns. But the PWCP can always find another doctor. When things get slow, another surgery can be lined up. Narcotics are always in order after another surgery. Nobody wants the pain, but some prefer the lifestyle. So be it.

The other choice or option is, of course, what this book encourages people who have chronic benign intractable pain to follow. It involves major change and a movement away from victimization. It involves taking responsibility, making a new commitment, sacrifice, guts, usually getting off drugs, starting an exercise program, practicing relaxation techniques, developing new eating habits, and entering group and family therapy. Perhaps the change entails an inpatient or outpatient stay in a chemical dependency or chronic pain unit, and hopefully, Chronic Pain Anonymous for a lifetime. This road of change for the PWCP, although not easy, is full of rewards. There's no promise of getting rid of 100% of the pain, but at least there's hope. The PWCP can have pride in attaining well-earned accomplishments. There's the admiration of friends and family who appreciate all the PWCP's efforts. There's always a Higher Power "directing traffic" and lending a helping hand. And there's a whole new world of undiscovered friends in CPA who stand ready to help. Making a change in your life is not a perfect road, but it is profoundly better than living your life as a victim.

The choice to be a victim is usually made easy for the PWCP, first by the pain itself, then by all the circumstances surrounding the pain lifestyle. In the following chapters and in Book II, the role of Chronic Pain Anonymous will be discussed in helping the PWCP embrace major change, become empowered, and leave behind the victim's fate.

# The Addict and the PWCP

▲   This book has noted the many similarities between an addict and the person suffering from chronic pain. If the two conditions are compared side by side, the characteristics are startling. Take a look:

| Addiction | Chronic Pain |
|---|---|
| Loss of Control | Loss of Control |
| Preoccupation | Preoccupation |
| Continued use despite adverse consequences | Continued negative conduct despite adverse consequences |
| Progression | Progression |

All *drinkers* are not out of control; only alcoholics lose control. Similarly, all PWCPs are not out of control; only those who are out of control need special help with their lives. Being out of control spells trouble: trouble at home, at work, and on the social front; being subjected to numerous surgeries with no relief; being hooked on multiple drugs; having no self-respect, money, friends, future, or family; talk about putting a gun in the mouth or taking a handful of pills to "end it all"; and exhausting all resources, medical and financial, and ending up worse than ever. Loss of control gets people into trouble, period.

One of the major characteristic traits found in people with chronic pain is preoccupation, and that also holds true for the addict. A PWCP goes to bed with pain and wakes up with pain; life revolves around pain. For the addict, life revolves around the abused substance. An addict keeps using until the grave, knowing full well where the addiction leads. Chronic benign intractable pain sufferers stick with the same conduct or behavior even though they, too, know where it's leading. Both the addict and the PWCP deny their problems. It's usually easy to pinpoint the addict's decline: the early, middle, or late stages of addiction usually depend on how much trouble has resulted. You could do the same evaluation for a person with chronic pain, too. The addict and the PWCP have both lost the ability to cope with their problems. And the comparison could go on.

Since the two conditions are so similar, shouldn't the same treatment that works for the alcoholic or any other drug addict work for someone with chronic benign intractable pain?

## What Works for Addicts

Once upon a time, addicts were locked up for several years to "treat" their addiction, but the results were poor. Through the years, a multidisciplinary approach evolved, culminating in an addict's lifelong involvement with an Anonymous support group. Some psychiatrists and psychologists claim that mental problems cause chronic pain, just as mental problems (such as depression) cause alcoholism and other addictions. As they see it, these mental difficulties are the result of too many or too few neurotransmitters being present in critical areas of a person's nervous system. The solution for some of these professionals is to prescribe medications which biochemically manipulate pain, mental problems, and so on. This is a simplistic explanation, obviously. Most professionals tend to offer anything they feel might help the problem of chronic pain or addiction, and most readily admit to frustrating failures. "Fixing" by professionals doesn't seem to work very well. "Fixing yourself," however, is a different consideration.

By far the best program that has come into being for the treatment of addiction is AA, Alcoholics Anonymous. Everything else pales by comparison. Since the 1930s, AA has been packing in addicts and offering simple, yet effective wellness tools. There are few towns in the United States without several AA meetings daily, and there are hundreds in any medium-sized city. AA is prolific because it works. It isn't perfect, but there's nothing better. It has saved millions of lives and will save many millions more. The philosophy of AA is simple, but not easy, and addicts who buy into it 100% usually turn out to be superb people. They don't just get well, they get "weller than well" as long as they work their program. It makes infinite sense to have the PWCP use it for pain management, too.

AA is based on Twelve Steps. Most good treatment programs in the United States are "Twelve Step Programs." It simply means that their philosophy and focus of treatment are AA-based. Not only does the Twelve Step program approach work, but it also leaves the patient with a follow-up, aftercare program that keeps meeting needs and resolving issues. On top of that, the aftercare doesn't cost anything but individual effort and time.

## The AA Model

AA is a self-help program—responsibility rests

with the individual. No one can do the work for someone else in the program, but people do help other people. Every AA member finds a good, solid sponsor whose duty it is to take serious charge of new members and guide them through the Twelve Steps. Most sponsors take their duties to heart, just like they take their programs. AA to them is a life or death situation, and they take the work seriously. That's not to say that AA members don't have a lot of fun, too. AA is not for morose, long-faced, pessimistic, doomsday kind of people. In fact, one of the things that attracts people to AA is the common denominator of people enjoying themselves. At first, visitors can't quite figure out why members are having such a good time. The friendly atmosphere tends to bring many of them back for more meetings. Enjoying life without drugs is a new experience for them.

Relapse in AA, unfortunately, is not unheard of. Some in the program never relapse. Some intrepid souls have to go back and do more research. Sometimes a slip back into addiction can be therapeutic, because people learn from their mistakes and nobody is perfect. Most take their beating and come back to AA with more humility. They listen harder and work their self-recovery program more diligently. The beautiful part about AA is that usually several other members have been over that same rough road and know how it feels. They realize that any addict, including themselves, can relapse, so there is no loss of face or respect. Members attend the meetings gaining strength from each other, and they always come away with something helpful.

Honesty and humility seem to be the key ingredients in AA. Members are all over each other when they notice they are less than honest. "Tough love" is sometimes hard on the ego, but honesty is what the program is all about. It's difficult to be phony when everyone else is striving to be honest. Humility is also a very high priority. Proud people are in for a rough ride.

AA meetings are like people. Sometimes they're good to wonderful; sometimes they aren't so great. AA members say that if they go to fifteen meetings, five will be terrific, five good, and five fair to poor. Most members have a "home group" but they move around. New faces, new ideas, and new locations add spice to the program. Mostly, AA is composed of very nice people doing their best to stay off drugs and alcohol. They're no brighter, no slower than you or others...they're just good people trying to stay straight.

Some people get the notion that AA is filled with "religious fanatics." AA is theistic in that as part of the Steps, members admit to a higher power outside themselves that can restore their sanity. The "Higher Power" can be the group process itself or a telephone pole, for that matter. Nobody shoves a specific concept of God down their throats. There are atheists in AA who get along just fine. The fact is that most AA members have drifted away from organized religion. When addiction set in, God was usually shoved out. Most eventually drift back in to some religious fold, but it's an individual decision. Religion and all other controversial subjects which might disturb the group, are left at the doorstep. AA endorses no organizations, they have no money, and they owe allegiance to no person or no special group. About the only qualification you need when showing up for a meeting is the sincere desire to stay off drugs and alcohol.

AA is a very loosely-knit organization. There are no generals, colonels, captains, sergeants, etc. Many business executives are dumbfounded to see that it works at all. The membership officers of AA are changed often and they understand their role is to serve the other members. There's no roll call. People come and go. The order of business depends on who is running the meeting that day, or what the *group* decides for protocol. There are no magnificent headquarters. A central office exists primarily for the distribution of information. AA members say the glue that keeps them all together is a quiet spirituality that seems to lack definition. It's a unique organization made up of very special and unique people.

## Walking the Talk

How people manage their addictions in AA is important to understanding chronic pain management, too. The Twelve Steps are the backbone of AA. When a person joins the group, he or she starts with the First Step and carefully takes each one in order, doing the work for each Step ("walking the talk") as if his life depends on it. Sponsors help, and other members pitch in when requested. From AA's inception, people have been trying to add, subtract, or modify the Twelve Steps, but they remain unaltered at present. Many other organizations have sprung up, all based on the original Steps. Today there's a Gamblers Anonymous, Sex Anonymous, Overeaters Anonymous, Narcotics Anonymous, Pills Anonymous, Parents Anonymous, Cocaine Anonymous, Alanon, and Alateen, just to name a few. All of these and many more use the Steps as a guide to turn their members' lives around. Why can't a person suffering from chronic intractable pain use the Twelve Steps to turn their lives around, too? Remarkable similarities exist between the addict and the PWCP, and it therefore seems logical to advocate for the start-up of a Chronic Pain Anonymous group. What does a PWCP have to lose? It wouldn't cost anything but time and effort, and it would help the PWCP bring more self-control and meaning back into life.

Chronic Pain Anonymous (CPA) would not be all things to all people. An estimated forty-five million Americans have chronic headaches, and seventeen million of them suffer from migraines. Sixty-five to seventy million Americans have some type of chronic pain. Not all of these people would need CPA. CPA is only for those who have exhausted the medical route with every other physician in town, been through a continuum of surgeries with little or no success, explored the pill route, and every other acceptable and unacceptable route with nothing to show but addiction and more bills. In other words, CPA is for people who are fed up with the merry-go-round of dysfunction. They'd like to see some progress for a change. They want to see a modicum of solid success.

There's little magic about the way men and women get into AA. AA members usually make their entrance after having been beaten up mentally and physically—but not without a furious fight. They've tried the other thousand ways to stop drinking and have failed miserably. Most have known about AA for years, but they have been expert in the use of denial and most wander around until they are half-dead before they swallow their pride and attend a meeting. Members don't show up for their first meeting because things are going well. They show up because they are losing their hold on life. They're sick, and most arrive at the Twelve Step doorway because there's nothing left. Families tell them to take a hike—wives, husbands, children, and all significant others have "had it." Their job is in jeopardy or lost, and most friends have waved the white flag. Everyone's simply become worn out with the addict's broken record of promises to change. People don't show up in treatment for laughs, either. Some crisis brings them in. Crises motivate them.

CPA is much the same as AA. If there was some magical "cure" for the pain, you can bet it has been tried and tried and tried. None exists, and pain is a cruel mistress. Members are likely to show up at a CPA meeting because there's little or no hope wherever they turn. Like the addict, PWCPs also wear out their families, their jobs are long gone, and their social lives are a thing of the past. They live with the pain and it steadily erodes their lives. They will not show up in CPA because they have nothing else to do. They will become interested in CPA because they're looking for a way out or a new approach—one *they* can do. With CPA they can be in the driver's seat, and they can be in control. No one will drag a PWCP into a CPA meeting kicking and screaming. If they're satisfied with the victim's lifestyle and all the dysfunction they have going on in their lives, then so be it. CPA doesn't recruit (neither does AA). People will come of their own volition. The only prerequisite is wanting help.

## Backsliding and CPA

Many people who are still drinking find themselves at AA meetings. As long as they're not disruptive, they're not tossed out. Many of them try to stop drinking and they try hard, but they just can't quite swing it. They quit for awhile, but fail, and some individuals seem to make a career of it. Some have to be "under the influence" to find the courage to walk into their first NA or CA meeting. Sanctity and purity is great to strive for in Twelve Step groups, but members are people and most people aren't perfect. Slips and backsliding happen, and they are regrettable and sometimes fatal. CPA members may do their share of backsliding, too.

There is little difference showing up at an AA meeting "three sheets to the wind" or waltzing into a CPA meeting "out of your mind" on pills. It's usually a waste of time inviting someone into group therapy when they're loaded on tranquilizers. The pills do most of the talking. In chemical dependency units, professionals usually wait until a patient is clean and off medication before allowing therapy. The reason is obvious: the counselor wants the patient operating on all of his or her own cylinders. There are exceptions, however, to this "pill rule." Some individuals need medications in order to function. There are mentally ill people who can't function without major tranquilizers. They need them to survive as much as a diabetic needs insulin.

Schizophrenics are aided by major tranquilizers such as thorazine, Mellaril, and other substances. There's not much gray area when major tranquilizers produce a profound, positive reaction in the conduct of these individuals. There's another large group of people with "affective" disorders. Most of them are diagnosed by mental health professionals as being "manic," "depressed," or "bipolar" (manic-depressive). They're prescribed drugs such as lithium or combinations of antidepressants. There's also much more gray area in this group, too. As a rule, if a mind-altering drug helps in overall functioning, it's wise to stick with it.

Mind-altering agents encompass most narcotics, tranquilizers, and sleeping pills. Non-steroid inflammatory agents are not mind-altering. Neither are products like aspirin or acetaminophen. Used intel-

ligently by the PWCP, these drugs are no problem.
Overuse is always trouble. Narcotics are different—
they're definitely mind-altering and not conducive to
the successful functioning of most PWCPs.

People with chronic pain may kick the pill habit in
treatment, but when they go home, the struggle is
incredible. When relief is only as far as the medicine
cabinet or a telephone call to the family doctor, it's
"white knuckle" time! All the hard work spent getting
off the drugs can be dissipated very quickly by one
lapse of concentration. PWCPs historically are not
rocks. Some, like many Anonymous members before
them, blow it. Should they be excluded from CPA
meetings? As long as they're not disruptive, they
should be included. As long as they're sincerely
trying, it would not be responsible or reasonable to
exclude them from help. As long as they're giving it
their best, they need a helping hand, and CPA is filled
with many helping hands.

Isn't it difficult for someone trying to stay abstinent from mind-altering drugs to associate with
another person who is using? This is a tough question. It's difficult to stay clean when in the presence
of others who choose to use drugs. Chronic pain
sufferers have about all they can handle dealing with
their own pain. When someone shows up at a CPA
meeting obviously on drugs, it isn't good for the
PWCPs who are sweating blood trying their best to
keep away from the "forbidden fruit." Wisdom and
patience are called for in dealing with such situations, but then all Anonymous groups have an ace in
the hole. It's called spirituality. AA, CPA, NA, CA, and
other Twelve Step support groups are all spiritual
programs. Spirituality involves much more than
prayer and mysticism. Spiritual "warmth" flows
among individuals in the meetings, and perhaps this

force provides the impetus to go the extra mile in coping with special situations. It usually works out and gives anyone who is backsliding a wellspring of loving support and encouragement from the other members.

Sadly, even physicians who are well aware of a patient's long history with chronic pain won't curtail or cut off narcotic prescriptions. As long as the PWCP can pay or has insurance, there's always someone around to furnish the pills. Some physicians truly continue to write these prescriptions because they think it's the humane thing to do. Others are just interested in cashflow. But the biggest factor is that a PWCP can generally manipulate most physicians. If they want the pills, they'll get them.

Alcohol and marijuana (plus all the other "street" or "recreational" chemicals) are mind-altering drugs. They turn the average person into a space cadet. A space cadet at a CPA meeting will accomplish little except rubbing other members the wrong way. These other substances are not high on the list in the pain-relieving medical armamentarium. Alcohol is by far the biggest offender. Pain is a great excuse to consume alcohol. When alcohol is combined with an analgesic there's a minimal synergistic effect, but over the long run, alcohol is absolutely worthless for pain. Showing up "blitzed" at a CPA meeting will not elevate the mood of other members who are trying to make major positive changes in their lives. Alcoholics are not famous for clear thinking when they drink. A CPA meeting requires a fully functioning, rested mind.

Tranquilizers are a monumental concern for the PWCP who would like to embrace the Twelve Steps. It seems that in our society it's difficult to find anyone who is not taking librium, valium, xanax, ativan, halcion, restoril, dalmane, serax, etc. Some people actually need them, but benzodiazepine addiction is a very tough detoxification. Pain creates stress and anxiety, stress and anxiety feed the pain, and anyone who has stress in their lives is offered tranquilizers. Headaches, backaches, ulcers, colitis, coronaries, insomnia, the bilateral tweets—just about anything—seems to require tranquilizers. PWCPs always have about twenty-five different reasons to get in line for them. Anxiety is the constant companion of chronic pain, tranquilizers are anxiolytics, and they eliminate anxiety. So what's the problem? The problem is addiction. Tolerance and withdrawal generally spell dependency. As tolerance develops, the quantity of the drug is increased. Instead of popping into a CPA meeting drunk on alcohol, the PWCP could show up semi-non compos mentis on pills. Some will combine the tranquilizers with the booze for an infinitely worse combination. Tranquilizers, all by themselves, are enough trouble.

Most sleeping pills are benzodiazepines. They're a plague to older people, and many chronic pain sufferers are elderly. When you age, sleep is not as sound. Older people tend to sleep lightly, awaken more often, and spend more time in bed lying awake. When a person lays in front of the TV for long periods of time, sleep will not happen at night. Lack of exercise (often excruciating for pain-sufferers) will promote sleeplessness. Sleeping pills are as easy to get as tranquilizers and have a similar result. When booze is considered too uncivilized, out come the pills. To compound the problem, many medications *cause* insomnia. Caffeine also interferes with rest.

At CPA, members will learn how to handle their sleep problems without benzodiazepines. Running around all fogged-up from the sleeping pills of the night before is not advised when a PWCP is trying to cope with chronic pain. A good mattress helps. PWCPs learn *not* to read, eat, write letters, or watch TV from bed. These behaviors create poor sleeping hygiene. They learn how important it is to develop regular sleep habits. Temperature control is also an important factor. CPA affords a forum to discuss these and other natural remedies.

# Forming a CPA Group

When several people with chronic benign intractable pain decide they want to start a Chronic Pain Anonymous group, they do. The only real qualification needed to attend an AA meeting is a sincere desire to stay off alcohol. The only real qualification needed to go to a CPA meeting is a sincere desire to learn *to live* with chronic pain. Does a PWCP ever get rid of the pain entirely? Probably not. Does an alcoholic ever stop becoming an alcoholic? Definitely not. The direct result is a different attitude and the acquisition of strength and encouragement from fellow members. Meetings provide an opportunity to share views and rub elbows with people who have similar problems. They give members a good shot at coping better with life in general.

AA meetings have been held almost anywhere. Elegant surroundings are nice, but hardly necessary. Any reasonable place where several people can sit and be able to talk will suffice. No one goes to a support group meeting for comfortable surroundings, although for Chronic Pain Anonymous it's a great idea to look for locations that accommodate wheelchairs and have barrier-free designs and restricted-access parking. People with chronic pain are not enthusiastic about climbing ten flights of stairs, either! In general, CPA meetings can be held at any reasonable, physically convenient location.

Every chronic pain management unit and every chemical dependency facility should host several meetings per week. These facilities usually have meeting space available and, of course, it offers a great excuse to get former patients back to the unit with regularity. CPA meetings boost census. Other patients with chronic pain are naturally drawn to the unit. The same is true of substance abuse units, of which there are thousands. All substance abuse treatment centers admit patients with chronic pain for narcotic and other mind-altering substance withdrawal. PWCPs feel quite different and relate poorly to the other patients without the pain factor, and post-treatment, they're not as comfortable in AA or other Anonymous meetings. Most PWCPs are encouraged to attend any Anonymous meeting available, but it would be best for the PWCP to come back to the same treatment facility for a CPA meeting. All it takes is a few energetic souls to start up a new group. Every substance abuse treatment center should have a CPA meeting several nights a week. Chronic pain sufferers can attend any Anonymous meeting, but they will do best at CPA meetings.

The protocol for CPA is the same as for any AA meeting. There should be no quandary about *how* meetings are conducted. New meetings of AA are always springing up. Any experienced AA member may offer direction and advice on how to start a CPA group, and all communities seem to have AA central offices. The yellow pages of the phone book usually list the AA central office numbers. Many qualified AA members would be only too willing to help anyone who makes a request to start up a CPA group. Most would consider it a privilege to be of service, affording them an opportunity to give back to others the direction and purpose in life that has been given to them. Setting up new CPA meetings may be an exciting project for them.

Chronic Pain Anonymous should proliferate. By virtue of the number of PWCPs, groups should never want for members. Any person with a sincere wish to cope with his or her pain should be welcome, and there are millions out there needing help. If chronic pain is destroying your home, work, or social life; if chronic pain is the cause of dysfunction in any part of your life; if chronic pain results in deep trouble of any sort in your daily activity, it's a good reason to seek out a CPA meeting. There's nothing quite like sharing your feelings, wants, experiences, hopes, fears, anxieties, knowledge, frustrations, anger, joys, and despair with others who have been traveling down the same road.

Everyone appreciates an opportunity to discuss problems with others who have had similar experiences. Soldiers who know the fears and frustrations of battle find solace and comfort discussing mutual problems with others who have been through trauma of the same nature. Vietnam vets are grateful to talk with other Vietnam vets. There's an immediate rapport. Understanding comes relatively easy among people of a common background. This is particularly true of people with chronic benign intractable pain.

People who suffer from chronic pain have special needs as well as problems. Narcotics Anonymous members attend AA when they can't find an NA meeting. Overeaters Anonymous members attend AA when they can't find an OA meeting. It's all the same Twelve Step philosophy. However, hardly without exception, all gravitate to their own organizations when meetings are accessible. They do so out of necessity.

People with chronic pain need to talk to other people with chronic pain. It's quite true that all Anonymous members have experienced *acute* pain, but few have a clue as to what constitutes the chronic condition. When people with chronic pain look for comfort and understanding, when PWCPs see the need to make significant behavioral changes in their lives, they need a room full of people who have chronic benign intractable pain. It makes a world of difference. And when the gathering is not just a "bull session," when the meeting is based on the principles and philosophy of AA, there's going to be major progress made.

When AA meetings get too large, they split off and start new AA meetings. When CPA meetings become too large, they will also split off into new CPA meetings. If a meeting gets to be overwhelming, members tend to pick up and go off to other meetings where they feel more comfortable. They just change their base of operations. People will go to where they feel most comfortable. Some meetings will feel wonderful and beneficial today, but tomorrow they may be a waste of time. Meetings are just like people—they're never quite the same. Almost without exception, however, members will come away with *something,* regardless of the quality of the meeting.

In AA they say, "bring the body, the mind follows." The same holds true for Chronic Pain Anonymous; just showing up helps, and soon your whole self with participate and become involved in the healing process. CPA is a lifetime support program for helping PWCPs live full and productive lives as they manage their chronic pain conditions. If you can't escape pain in your everyday reality—if you truly must *live with pain*— the modalities covered in Book I, along with Chronic Pain Anonymous, should be your tools to break the stranglehold pain has put on every aspect of your life. ▲

# Book II

## Chronic Pain Anonymous

# The Foundations

▲   Tremendous strides have been made over the past twenty to thirty years in the field of pain physiology. A host of brilliant scientists have devoted their lives to the study of this ubiquitous, fascinating phenomenon, trying to unveil the mysteries of pain. Over the last few decades more knowledge and understanding about pain has surfaced than over the last thousand years:

• We can now trace pain (with reasonable certitude) from receptors in the periphery—skin, muscle, fascia, bones, etc.—through pathways into the spine and up the spinal cord, and then track impulses through the myriad of intricate nerve tissue to specific destinations in the brain.

• We are gaining in knowledge about how the brain and spinal cord respond and modify pain. We know which nerves carry pain impulses, and at what speed; we know the various types of receptors in the periphery and how they function.

• We now have a pretty good idea of how many of the billion neurons in the central nervous system are regulated and influenced by neurochemicals called neurotransmitters.

• We are learning how to manipulate these neurotransmitters to modify pain.

• We have learned how to stimulate nerves outside the central nervous system electronically to modify pain.

• We have developed surgical techniques that, in specific cases, may eliminate pain completely.

But we have come a million miles in the field and still feel helpless when faced with what we do not know. Our subject is chronic benign intractable pain—the pain that doesn't go away. It baffles the experts, and cripples the lives of People With Chronic Pain (PWCPs), their family, friends, and co-workers.

## Problem

It's a fact that millions of people continue to suffer with pain day in and day out, spend billions of dollars trying to get some help, and find no relief. Americans spend over $80 billion every year for temporary pain relief, everything from pills to heating pads. Somewhere along the mysterious six-month line they crossed from acute to chronic pain, and they have no alternative but to learn to live with it. Somehow their pain became locked up in the central nervous system, and no medication, no surgery, and no special technique will dislodge it. People with chronic pain must accept the fact they have a "tiger by the tail." They must learn to control pain before it controls them and ruins their lives in the process.

## Acute Pain

For good reason, most of us do not appreciate acute pain. Hurt is something we try to avoid assiduously. Acute pain is not all bad, however. Pain provides a vital service: it lets us know something is wrong. If you break a leg, there is pain; you are not about to use that leg. The pain is a loud and clear message to stop walking. Exposure to fire causes terrible pain; if you did not experience pain, you would allow further damage to your tissue. If you experience chest pain, you pull up short; if pain did not give a warning that a portion of your heart muscle was deprived of blood, it could easily mean the difference between life or death. In conditions where the pain mechanism is knocked out, such as diabetic neuropathy or leprosy, terrible tissue damage often occurs without the suffering person even knowing.

## Chronic Pain

Beyond that "watch-dog" role, chronic pain has not much redeeming value. It forces people to become exceptional, if they're able to rise above the pain. That's admirable. Also, fighting chronic pain twenty-four hours a day and winning the contest certainly develops unusual character. But, let's face it, PWCPs are tested to their limits; chronic pain hasn't much to offer that is a plus.

Some people with chronic pain are somehow able to subjugate it sufficiently so it does not interfere with their lives. They are a rare breed. Whether they just turn it all over to God or their Higher Power and grit their teeth or just miraculously learn to cope, no one knows. However, the huge majority of chronic pain sufferers are searching for any relief they can find and are willing to pay any price for it, financially, physically, spiritually—whatever it takes. They're willing to go to any length to get some relief.

## Chronic Pain vs. Addiction

Over the past twenty-four years of full-time work

with alcoholics, drug addicts, and PWCPs, I have noticed rather remarkable similarities between people suffering from chronic pain and those addicted to a variety of drugs. (Alcohol by the way, is by far the most abused drug.)

Both the addict and the PWCP have somehow acquired an intractable, devastating problem that could eventually destroy them. Both are heavily into denial. Both have normally exhausted every resource before admitting their problem. Both have looked for a cure, a "magic bullet," for years. Both have become worn out searching for something outside of themselves to fix the problem. Both tend to blame God for giving them such an inordinate burden. Both become extremely depressed, and rightly so. Both are highly prone to relapse. Both tend to fail unless they have involved significant others in their lives, and in their families. Both must make substantial lifestyle changes.

Chronic pain sufferers and addicts must learn to enjoy life; break free from their shells; exercise daily; eat balanced meals; and avoid sugar, stimulants, pain-killing drugs, alcohol, sleeping pills, excesses of all kinds, etc. Both never recover, but they can enter a state of recovering. Both must accept a life sentence of commitment. If they stick with their self-management programs, both parties tend to turn into exceptional human beings.

## Similarities

In my experience, most people suffering from chronic pain have a very difficult time seeing the similarity between themselves and drug addicts. They tend to look down their noses at addicts and alcoholics. After all, they think, those people are weak-willed, self-centered, instant-gratification types who voluntarily exposed themselves to dangerous drugs while seeking pleasure. Somehow, along the way, they got hooked in the process. Chronic pain sufferers, on the other hand, feel they ended up with their problem through no fault of their own. If they eventually became dependent on drugs, it was the fault of some doctor who was too free with the prescription pad. It wasn't their fault! The drug addict asked for it, but they didn't. (In reality, they're wrong about the addict/alcoholic. I have never met an addict who purposely set out to end up that way. I've never met an alcoholic who purposely wanted to live life as a drunk.)

In general, however, it seems most people feel that resisting alcoholism and drugs is merely a matter of willpower. People have been telling me for years that alcoholics and other drug addicts are just "weak-willed." (Some of those same people tend to say the same about PWCPs—no willpower! I usually tell these critics that the next time they get diarrhea, just use willpower. It makes about as much sense.) Once pain gets locked into the central nervous system, once the drug abuser crosses the nebulous line, forget about willpower. From then on, it's a matter of working on a constant, uplifting, lifelong program to avoid a life of abject misery that could destroy them and adversely affect everyone around them.

## Depression

Depression seems to come with the territory for a PWCP. When you are depressed, you feel hopeless and helpless. Chronic pain patients have every reason to feel that way. A terrible problem is eating them alive. Their pain is factored into every equation concerning any major decision. Often there may be no money, home, work, or social life. Life with chronic pain leads you to think life isn't worth living. Your self-esteem is poor. You begin to entertain thoughts about how good it would be to be out of all of it. You become paralyzed with fear, you can't concentrate, and you have trouble sleeping and eating. Your energy level is nil. These are classical signs of depression, and they're classically found in PWCPs and addicts alike.

## Treatment Centers

Many a PWCP ends up seeking treatment in a rehabilitation center for withdrawal from narcotics, tranquilizers, or alcohol, or any combination of substances. They don't relate very well in treatment, and they all have one common complaint: "Sure, you take me off my pills, and then what the hell am I going to do for my pain?" Perfectly healthy drug addicts experience pain when withdrawn from narcotics; the PWCP will also experience the usual withdrawal symptoms, plus an increase in the level of pain. (This is a difficult enough phase in a good, supportive clinical environment. Outpatients don't fare well because they need constant encouragement and reinforcement from others.) Once withdrawal is accomplished, however, the PWCP is often pleasantly surprised to find the pain stabilizes at a tolerable level. This is particularly true if other modalities have been introduced into the withdrawal phase, such as physical therapy, TENS units, a balanced diet, an exercise program, relaxation techniques, and so on.

The challenge really begins when it comes time to leave the treatment facility. Most PWCPs still feel like fish out of water. They have trouble relating to an alcoholic even if they're alcoholics themselves! Narcotic addicts tend to use illegal drugs, and a person with chronic pain uses prescription drugs. They can try "Pills Anonymous," but many in this Anonymous group are not chronic pain patients. With no place to call home, PWCPs tend to relapse quickly.

# Aftercare

From a pragmatic perspective, there is no big difference between treatment and aftercare for people suffering from chronic pain and those suffering from drug addiction. Alcoholics and other drug addicts have numerous options for treatment, and a built-in post-treatment support system that's hard to beat. A support system costs nothing but time and effort. Treatment centers seem to be on every street corner today, if you have insurance or are willing to pay the fees. The post-treatment support system is available everywhere. In my city of 600,000, there must be at least 300 to 400 such groups: Alcoholics Anonymous (AA), Narcotics Anonymous, Cocaine Anonymous, Al Anon, Alateen, Codependency Anonymous, Sex Anonymous, Gambler's Anonymous—you-name-it Anonymous! They're all based on the principles and philosophy of Alcoholics Anonymous which was founded in the 1930s. (A priest friend of mine suggests that these principles must have been divinely inspired. He's not a member himself, but he's perceptive and wise, and I suspect there's a good deal of truth in his observation.)

# Chronic Pain Management Units

Chronic pain management units, however, are few and far between. Insurance companies have been historically opposed to medical reimbursement for this type of treatment. Interestingly enough, when I opened a Substance Dependency Unit in 1969, the same tough attitude existed for alcohol and other substance abuse treatment. Insurance companies always paid one way or another in those days, however, because alcoholics ended up hospitalized with other "acceptable" diagnoses.

When the insurance climate changed, treatment centers flourished. Perhaps some day the same will be true for chronic pain management units. Some do exist, and they perform excellent work, but you must look for them. They address pain management through group and individual therapy. They rely heavily on occupational and physical therapy and use biofeedback and relaxation techniques. Some offer TENS units, nerve blocks, ice massage, and osteopathic manipulation, and they involve the entire family, if possible. You could hardly graduate from three to four weeks of this concentrated therapy and not leave in a much improved status.

## Predicament

The problem for the PWCP is that there's no universal, cheap, efficient, and proven system of aftercare like the program AA offers alcoholics. The PWCP acquires great new tools, a new outlook on life, is off all narcotics, is able to do physical tasks that before were unthinkable and yet, unless he or she lives next door to the hospital and can afford professional aftercare, their support system is gone. Most relapse quickly. Gains are rapidly dissipated and the money invested in recovery is wasted.

A good support system is needed to enforce the use of newly-acquired recovery tools. Support from others is essential. Strength from peers who have been over the same road must be drawn upon. A program with a first-rate track record based on a substantial, proven philosophy must be available for the PWCP's recovery to continue.

# Quality

Just as people with drug problems "made it" for centuries without special treatment centers, many PWCPs "make it" without first going through special chronic pain management units. People stayed sober before AA-based groups existed, but not at the same rate or with the same quality of life. People are impressed by the quality of sobriety attained by the membership of these groups. "White-knuckle" sobriety is a great achievement, but you can be sober and still be miserable. Practicing the principles and philosophy of AA gives good quality-of-life sobriety.

## Chronic Pain Anonymous

Chronic pain management units or substance abuse treatment centers can be invaluable; they give a solid foundation for physical recovery. Still, there's a great need for a solid, inexpensive support system for aftercare. What happens when there's no after-care program, no supportive group catering to the particular problems associated with chronic pain? What happens to the person with limited financial resources who can't afford to go to professional pain management facilities?

Just as in AA, NA, or any Anonymous organization, chronic pain sufferers should be able to simply walk in off the street and ask for help. There should be a place for them, and there is! It's called *Chronic Pain Anonymous.*

# Support

Chronic Pain Anonymous— What's in a name?

I suspect most people who are searching for a support group for chronic pain have only one prerequisite for joining: to stop the addiction process. You must want to get off the merry-go-round.

What PWCPs need is an AA-based group tailored to their specific needs. What to call it?

The name Chronic Pain Anonymous seems to make sense. Let's face it, very few people have first-hand knowledge of what chronic pain is all about. Most people *think* they do. They know and understand acute pain because just about everyone has experienced it. Chronic pain, however, is something very different. When someone with chronic pain tries to explain the terrible and constant hurt, the routine response is, "Yeah, I had that once, I know exactly how you feel!" They have no inkling! The closest you can come to finding someone who understands the misery of chronic pain is relating to another person who has been down a similar road.

## Empathy

You can't quantify pain. It doesn't come in inches, yards, pounds, or kilograms. Even describing pain can be difficult. Only with sensitive, sophisticated probing can you come away with a reasonable idea of how much someone else hurts. Our mental, emotional, social, ethnic, and even religious backgrounds play a large part in how we handle pain. Pain is extremely complicated, but people who have had similar experiences tend to relate. They understand, and in a support group they share knowledge and love and keep each other "straight." They become buddies. They become pals, "pain pals."

## Alcoholics Anonymous

Every group needs structure. Every business functions better with rules and regulations; otherwise, chaos takes over. Ideas, goals, rules, and ways of doing business are often "borrowed" from successful organizations. Why reinvent the wheel? The more successful the organization, the more likely the emulation. There must be more than fifty organizations that have evolved from AA. Chronic Pain Anonymous follows suit. Anyone who is able to assimilate the principles and philosophy of AA can't help but be better for the experience. There are already many PWCPs in Alcoholics Anonymous and Narcotics Anonymous because many PWCPs become addicted to narcotics, and some are on both alcohol and narcotics.

## Pills and Chronic Pain

Many PWCPs end up in substance abuse programs because they become addicted to the narcotics they use to control chronic pain. These patients are difficult to treat, because they usually maintain the attitude that if they stop the narcotics they won't be able to deal with their pain. Invariably they think withdrawal is too fast, and then they seek more medication. A PWCP who is hooked on drugs is difficult to withdraw because the withdrawal itself will exacerbate the chronic pain. The narcotics may have been prescribed in good faith, but people in withdrawal don't look kindly toward the physician who wrote the prescriptions. And every subsequent surgery will mean another fight with the narcotics. The battle never seems to end.

## Common Denominator

CPA meetings are patterned after other Anonymous groups. You only need to substitute the word "chronic pain" for "alcohol" or "cocaine" or "heroin" or "sex" or "gambling." There is one common denominator that ties all AA-based recovery groups together: rarely does a person attend a meeting and not come away richer.

## Need

PWCPs need a special support group where they can let it all hang out. They need a support group where understanding abounds, love flows freely, knowledge is shared, drugs are off limits, and humor is explored—a support group where peers help keep each other straight. Each person needs to accept responsibility for getting well, and each PWCP needs an atmosphere that consists of other people striving to get well. CPA is an organization where they can leave their depression on the doorstep, where they can focus on self-esteem, and be able to laugh and cry in a comfortable environment with peers who understand them. PWCPs must learn to have fun again, to enjoy food again, to function again as productive members of their families and society. Sounds almost like "pie in the sky?"

Well, I've been witnessing people turn their lives around for over twenty-four years, just by using the principles and philosophy of AA. PWCPs can do the same. It won't be easy, as few things worthwhile are easy. It will involve a lot of time and effort. You must work AA's Twelve Steps, find a good sponsor, help others, and get outside of yourself. It takes time.

The main thing to do is just show up. There are several sayings in AA: "Bring the body and the mind follows!" "Keep coming back, it works!" and "Keep it simple!" Yes, there's usually something for everyone.

## The Steps

From this foundation of support for PWCPs, we can review the Twelve Steps as they apply to chronic pain.

# The Twelve Steps
## for Chronic Pain

### ▲ STEP 1

We admitted we were powerless over pain—that our lives had become unmanageable.

**The Foundation**

Every now and then we see a house that seems to be falling apart way before its time. Chances are the foundation is faulty. The best building won't stand up over time when placed on a shaky foundation. In education, we can't progress from one level to another without a proper foundation. We don't jump from grade school to college. We don't start post-graduate school without first completing under-graduate work. Step 1 needs to be approached in this manner, too. It's the foundation upon which the others lie.

**Importance**

Each Step is very important, but recovery begins with this one. Work on it must be thorough, it must be honest, and it must be good. I have known many people in AA who have done Step 1 regularly. Many sponsors insist this step is so important that they make their charges do this Step several times. They feel that if someone fails in the program, the major flaw is in a weak First Step.

## Powerlessness

The first hurdle the PWCP must get over is realizing that pain is eroding, if not destroying, his or her life. If the problem is "not that bad," the effort expended will be halfhearted. "Why fix something if it ain't broke?"

"Powerless over pain"—that's difficult to admit if you are a very proud person. Pride generally scuttles the program. It's not difficult to see proud people sabotage themselves, senselessly conning, kidding, and playing games with themselves until it's too late. Powerlessness equals defeat, they think. Many a proud person dies before becoming willing to admit defeat. Powerlessness means surrender, and pride will not allow surrender. It takes a humble person to admit pain is somehow locked up in their central nervous system and nothing, nothing is going to get rid of it. No PWCP wants to hear this, much less admit it.

You have to be a strong person to admit to powerlessness over pain, and you must really mean it. It must come from your heart. Talk is cheap.

## Unmanageability

To admit that your life has become unmanageable demands abject honesty. Two words that keep coming up constantly when doing Step 1 are "honesty" and "humility," qualities not easy for a person with chronic pain to have. If pride doesn't get in the way, dishonesty frequently does. People full of pride want to run their own show. Running their own show has gotten them nowhere, but they're not about to admit it. You must become honest to overcome pride. It's easy to philosophize and it's easy to talk. Being honest is another matter. Honest and humble people are able to admit pain is eating them alive, turning them into empty shells, and destroying any semblance of a normal life. Most continue to hold out for the "magic bullet," the miraculous cure that will eliminate their chronic pain. Most do not want to be told their only real hope lies within themselves.

## Superficiality

Superficiality has no place in Step 1, but it's a common pitfall. Many feel that failure in the program stems from a superficial First Step. A "good" First Step is absolutely exhausting, mentally and physically taxing. When people finish an excellent First Step, they say they feel as though they've been put through the wringer. Superficiality is concerned with the understanding of only the easily apparent and obvious. A superficial Step 1 wastes not only the time of the person giving it but also those listening to it. You must attack Step 1 with the total honesty that rarely encompasses the obvious and easily apparent. Soul-searching is a tough, mean business. There's no room for superficiality.

## Put It In Print

If at all possible, Step 1 should be written down. It's easier to gloss over, minimize, alter, fabricate, or delete when delivering this Step off the top of your head. Putting it in writing forces you to give it more thought, be more factual, and more honest. It helps to crystallize thought. The people who listen to it will not be literary critics. They're not interested in your syntax or grammar. They're looking for honesty, humility, and sincerity of feelings. Anything less from you is phony and second-rate. Putting Step 1 in print makes success more probable.

## Time

There are no hard and fast rules about how or when the First Step is given. Generally it's read by the individual doing the Step to peers. It's read to a group. This seems to work better because it affords immediate feedback, and groups tend to be much more up front and honest than on a one-to-one basis. If the effort is feeble, if the person giving it isn't sincere, if it's delivered with no feeling (in short, if it's superficial), the reader is confronted posthaste! Most of the time it's a heartwarming experience. The reader feels great, the group supportive, and the atmosphere is charged. When it's not so great, the speaker is often asked to do some or all of it over again. The proud become combative; the humble take another crack at it in the near future.

## Defense Mechanisms

There are some serious mental defense mechanisms that need to be discussed before launching headlong into the First Step. It helps to review them so they don't get in the way. Unless pointed out, they tend to mess up the process. With chronic pain, they may be even more important to recognize and tackle. If you keep these stumbling blocks in mind, you will be less apt to let them get in the way.

## Delusion and Denial

Loss of control automatically leads to powerlessness and unmanageability. Chronic pain readily causes loss of control in your life. Pain takes over your life just like heroin, cocaine, or alcohol does. You're no longer in charge; pain is, and it runs everything. When your life revolves around pain, when every waking moment and every decision is influenced by pain, then your life is out of control. So often this fact is very obvious to everyone except the person with the problem.

## Parallel

It's interesting to parallel an out-of-control PWCP to someone fighting the disease of alcoholism. Over 100 million Americans consume alcohol, and somewhere around fifteen million become alcoholics. Once they cross the line from use to abuse and dependency, their lives disintegrate. There's no family, no money, no pleasure, no self respect, no love—just a downward spiral until death. When alcoholics cross the line, they've lost control. When pain takes over and life begins to fall apart, similar things happen to the PWCP.

## Denial

Denial is the act of refusing to believe a fact. Doubling your normal weight and refusing to face the fact that you have a serious weight problem is denial. Refusing to accept cancer in a dying patient with documented disease—that's denial. Refusing to admit to a heroin or cocaine problem when looking at prison time, financial ruin, and constant physical harm—that's denial. Living as a recluse, dependent on pain medication, alienating your family and friends, no job, no prospects, no money, relentlessly seeking a phantom, miraculous cure—that's denial, too!

## Delusion

Delusion is a false belief. It means a belief in something contrary to fact. Objective evidence is ignored. Delusion allows you to dwell in a fantasy land. "Nothing is wrong with me. I just use a little too much medication now and then." "So I've had ten surgeries! The eleventh will take my pain away." "I don't have time for any damn meetings." "With all the new technology today, something will surely come along to eliminate my pain. It's just a matter of time." "My life isn't that bad. I'm strong! I'm in control, not the pain." "I'm not like you people. My life is not unmanageable." Delusions run rampant in the addiction population, and they're probably even more prominent in people suffering from chronic pain.

## Rationalization

Typically, rationalization allows you to devise superficial or plausible explanations or excuses for your actions, beliefs, and desires. It seems the more intellectual the person (either factual or imagined), the more likely this defense mechanism comes into play. "I'm not really an addict because my doctor prescribes for me." "I can't leave the house because I can't drive." "I can't walk well enough." "I'm afraid I'll fall." "I can't exercise. It makes my pain worse." "You get rid of my pain, then I'll get rid of my pills." "I'll join a support group if I can get permission from my husband, my son, my daughter, my surgeon . . . ." The run-of-the-mill PWCP may come up with five excuses; the so-called intellectual with chronic pain will come up with ten. Some are amazingly inventive.

## One-to-One vs. Group

Rationalization allows you to use your reasoning to stay sick. I suspect most of the time the PWCP doesn't see how very faulty and phony the reasoning is. On a one-to-one basis rationalization is very difficult to dislodge.

In a group of people with similar problems, challenging rationalizations is much easier to do and much more effective. Pride and lack of honesty are likely to surface. Rationalization is one tough customer and any PWCP, or any addict for that matter, may have become a black belt, world-class protagonist in its use.

Peers in a support group have traveled down the same road. They readily see what goes on. They've been there. They understand that going for the throat usually doesn't work. If such an approach had been used on them, they are much more likely, as a result, to use a kinder, gentler way of getting the job done. They understand how easy it is to give a PWCP reason to run. They are also very likely to have had trouble with authority figures because they've been burned, too. It's extremely easy to get locked in mental combat one-to-one, but in a group of peers it's much less likely.

## Formidable Wall

Rationalization is the brick and mortar people so often use to build a formidable wall around themselves, and God help anyone who tries to breech that wall! Often, by the time PWCPs seek help, they have lost amateur standing when it comes to explaining their conduct. A good CPA support group will not allow rationalization for a second. Half the group will probably react to this defense mechanism, almost by reflex. Most have used the same illogical excuses themselves, so they can point it out seven different ways without being insulting. (Professionals in the chronic pain management business often lack patience and sometimes with good reason. It's a tough business!) Peers tend not to "blow each other away." More often their patience seems infinite because they have been there.

Rationalization seems automatically to dissolve with time and effort. All you have to do is bring your body to the meetings. Soon, you will begin to see how very destructive your thinking has been, particularly when you begin to recognize the same conduct in others. Rationalization pops up at every meeting. Having it pointed out by several people makes it more palatable and acceptable. Few people wandering this world do not rationalize on a daily basis; for the most part, the rationalizations are wrong, but fairly harmless. When rationalization allows PWCPs to stay ill, however, it's no longer harmless. It's deadly.

## Projection

Projection is the unconscious act or process of ascribing to others your own ideas, impulses, or emotions, especially when they are undesirable or cause anxiety. This doesn't exactly sparkle with mental health. It's fairly hard to stop if it's an unconscious act; when you don't realize you're projecting, there's little you can do about it. In CPA, the group process can point to sick ideas, impulses, or emotions and wave a red flag.

## Shifting of Responsibility

Projection allows you to shift responsibility. Blame gets dumped on someone else. We all do it to some extent, and we all know these six most dreaded words: "It didn't happen on my shift!" When the PWCP allows projection to keep him or her sick, it has to be addressed or there will be no semblance of wellness. Projection has to be exposed and it has to be eradicated.

## Anger and Hostility

Anger, and frequently hostility, are mental bedfellows in chronic pain. It's difficult for anyone in chronic pain not to be seething with anger and filled with hostility. It's hard to imagine how someone who wakes up every morning in great pain, struggles all day long always in pain, performing tasks most people take for granted, could not be loaded with anger, unwittingly dumping hostility on the closest person around (usually a loved one) or something "out there" they hold responsible.

When doing Step 1, anger and hostility are likely to come up regularly, and unless checked, they can keep you miserable. If recognized, something can be done about them. If you don't pick up these culprits when preparing your First Step, they commonly come up when you present the Step to a group. Projection is a deadly type of mental virus. It drives people away. Unchecked it can be devastating. It wears those who care about you down to a frazzle. As time progresses, even the most stout-hearted get fed up and leave the PWCP to wallow in misery and self-pity. It's a hard scene to watch. The saddest aspect of projection is that the PWCP is often unaware of it.

## Repression and Suppression

To repress means to force the ideas and impulses of your painfully conscious mind into the unconscious. Repression is the mechanism by which your ideas and impulses are buried in your unconscious mind. To suppress means to consciously dismiss from your mind unacceptable ideas and impulses. Another saying at AA is that one is as sick as his or her secrets. Psychotherapists make their living dealing with repressed and suppressed mental material. Priests spend a good part of their lives dealing with this subject matter in the confessional. Not dealing with your "dirty linen" keeps you mentally unhealthy—cleaning the attic and then keeping it clean leads to great mental health.

## Mental Garbage

The First Step, properly done, forces a responsible look at all sorts of past and present conduct that most of us would prefer to ignore. More often than not, PWCPs have a ton of mental garbage that they would much prefer to just let be. Many take the position that they have enough physical pain to deal with. Why take on another burden of mental pain? They don't understand yet that such repressed, suppressed, and secretive garbage influences their physical pain. "As sick as your secrets" takes on new meaning. The First Step can get to be tumultuous; the more thoroughly done, the more you begin to realize how sick you have become physically and mentally. A professional counselor in a chronic pain management unit can be of immense value in dealing with suppressed material; most psychologists and psychiatrists do it for a living. A good sponsor may come riding to the rescue when suppressed and repressed material is confronted, but the process is sometimes tricky and sometimes needs professional attention. If someone in the clergy is familiar with the Twelve Steps and understands the process and philosophy, he or she can be extremely helpful. Seek help wherever it's available.

## Hostility and Humility

The two key words in the First Step are "powerlessness" and "unmanageability." The next two key words are "honesty" and "humility." People suffering from chronic pain cannot stray too far if they keep these words up front. The following format is merely a suggestion or a guide that may help you achieve a memorable First Step.

## First Step Presentation

I. Autobiography

The autobiography should contain a thumbnail sketch of your life. It should include the following:

A. Childhood (through preteen years)

1. Quality of relationship with parents and siblings

2. Earliest recollections of feelings about yourself

3. Early triumphs and significant losses

4. Religious influences in family

5. Attitudes in family about alcohol and/or other drugs

6. Attitudes in family about male/female roles in the family

B. Teen Years

1. Relationship with parents
2. Parents' relationship with each other
3. Major values passed on from parents
4. Attitude and performance in school
5. Attitude and performance in extra-curricular activities
6. Attitude about male/female relationships
7. Social network, dating, etc.
8. Feelings about yourself during this stage
9. Significant losses or failures during this period
10. Experimentation with any drugs (alcohol included)

C. Early Adult Life

1. Passage into adulthood
2. Ongoing relationships with parents, brothers, and sisters
3. Military experience
4. Social network
5. Marriage, separations, and divorce
6. Feelings about yourself during this stage
7. Education and career direction
8. Significant successes and/or failures
9. Alcohol or other drug use

D. Adult Life

1. Ongoing relationships with parents, sisters, and brothers
2. Career successes/failures
3. Outcome of goals
4. Marriage, separations, and divorce
5. Relationships with own children
6. Social relationships
7. Feelings about yourself during this stage
8. Significant successes and/or failures

9. Alcohol or other drug use

10. When your pain problem developed

E. Present—ask yourself:

1. How I view myself

2. How I view society and the world I live in

3. How I perceive other people view me

4. How I believe others view my chronic pain problem

II. Unmanageability

A. What does unmanageability mean to me?

B. Is my life unmanageable as a result of chronic pain?

C. How has chronic pain affected my social life?

1. Have I lost friends?

2. Do I now avoid certain people?

3. Have I alienated family members?

4. Have I become socially isolated?

5. What are three examples of how my social life has been affected by my chronic pain?

D. My physical condition

1. How do I view my general health?

2. Do I have trouble sleeping?

3. Do I use antacids for an upset stomach?

4. Do I lack energy?

5. Do I have constipation and/or diarrhea?

6. Have I deteriorated in body tone and physical appearance?

7. Have I gained or lost weight?

8. Have physicians tried to cut down on my medications?

9. Do I withhold accurate information about the quantity of analgesic drugs prescribed by my physicians?

10. What are three examples of how chronic pain has affected me physically?

E. What effect has chronic pain had on my financial status?

1. Have I made poor investments?
2. Have I overspent?
3. Am I in debt?
4. Have I mismanaged household funds?
5. Do I have any savings for my retirement?
6. Does my chronic pain problem override good judgment in financial matters?
7. Have I lost any jobs, promotions, etc. because of chronic pain?
8. What are three examples of how chronic pain has affected me financially?

F. What are direct-cost estimates of how much my chronic pain problem has cost me (in terms of dollars)?

1. Hospital costs
2. Physician costs
3. Drugs purchased
4. Legal fees (divorces, DUI's or citations for driving under the influence, lawsuits over injuries, etc.)
5. Lost jobs and promotions
6. Miscellaneous costs

G. How do my monthly expenditures for chronic pain stack up with costs for essentials (food, rent, utilities, etc.)?

H. What is the total percentage of my income spent on my pain problem?

I. My Job—my chronic pain has caused:

1. Lowered productivity?
2. Poor decision making?
3. Promotions passed over?
4. Absenteeism?
5. Conflicts with peers?
6. Disciplinary measures?
7. Termination?

8. Early retirement?
9. Feelings of guilt about quantity/quality of work?
10. Confrontation by colleagues?
11. What are three examples of how my chronic pain has interfered with my job or profession?
J. My home life
1. Do I perform well in household matters?
2. Do I accomplish daily chores?
3. Do I pay enough attention to my children's emotional, physical, and safety needs?
4. Do I eat with the family and prepare meals adequately and on time?
5. Do I engage in conflicts with the children over my pain problem?
6. Has my pain problem resulted in conflicts for family members amongst themselves?
7. How much TV do I watch?
8. Have I lost interest in family, hobbies, etc.?
9. Do I miss appointments/commitments?
10. What are three examples of how chronic pain has interfered with my household or parental responsibilities?
K. My retirement
1. Did I retire before I was financially able?
2. Did I fall short of my dreams about retirement?
3. Have I lost interest in hobbies or activities?
4. Have I become socially isolated?
5. Am I compromised financially?
6. Do I focus on the past more than I should?
7. What are three examples of how chronic pain has affected my retirement?
L. My values (What specific values have changed?)
1. Have I passed any bad checks?
2. Have I engaged in any sexual activities outside of marriage?

3. Have I become extremely emotional, hostile, or violent?

4. Have I physically or emotionally abused my spouse or children?

5. Have I lost interest in my physical appearance or personal hygiene?

6. Have I deprived my family of love and support?

7. Have I lied to my family, friends, or employer?

8. Have I contemplated or attempted suicide?

9. What are five examples of how chronic pain has caused me to alter my values?

M. My spiritual life

1. Has my chronic pain caused me to feel empty?

2. Have I moved more and more toward agnosticism as my chronic pain has taken over?

3. Do I feel abandoned by God?

4. Have I become hostile toward organized religion?

5. Have I stayed away from church because of guilt?

6. What are three examples of how chronic pain has affected my spiritual life?

N. My emotional problems

1. Do I feel depressed?

2. Do I think I am going crazy?

3. Do I think others are against me?

4. Do I have feelings of low self-esteem?

5. Do I fear social situations?

6. Do I lack intimacy?

7. Do I have difficulty getting close to other people?

8. Do I exhibit rigid thinking and intolerance with others?

9. Am I easily outraged?

10. Do I have temper tantrums?

11. Do I panic easily?

12. Do I harbor unexplained fears?

13. Do I feel lonely most of the time?
14. Do I have guilt feelings?
15. Do I feel a sense of impending doom?
16. Do I have vivid nightmares?
17. Do I have rapid mood swings?
18. Have I ever contemplated suicide?
19. What are five examples of how chronic pain has affected my emotional life?
   O. My sexual being
1. Do I have trouble getting and maintaining an erection, or ejaculating?
2. Do I have orgasms?
3. Have I lost interest in sex?
4. Has my partner lost interest in sex?
5. Have I become sexually promiscuous?
6. What are three examples of how chronic pain has affected my sex life?
   P. My life goals
1. Has chronic pain kept me from accomplishing my life goals?
2. Has it interfered with my education?
3. Has it kept me from entering a field or profession?
4. Has it interfered with advancement in a career?
5. Has chronic pain interfered with development of marital/family relationships?
6. Has chronic pain hampered my ability to find a spouse to share my life?
7. Am I able to put plans and ideas into action?
8. Do I frequently change goals? Do I often scatter my efforts?
9. Do I lack career motivation?
10. What are three examples of how chronic pain has interfered with my goals?
   Q. My family problems
1. Have I been verbally abusive to my family?

2. Have I been emotionally abusive to them?

3. Have I been physically abusive to them?

4. Have I lost the closeness I once felt?

5. Do I have the feeling that my family has lost respect for me?

6. Do I feel isolated in my family?

7. Am I an effective parent? Have I lost control of my children?

8. Has my spouse taken to using alcohol or other drugs more than usual?

9. Do I have extreme feelings of guilt or remorse?

10. Do I feel as though no one in the family understands me?

11. Am I withdrawing from family activities?

12. Am I separated from my family?

13. Am I divorced?

14. What are three examples of how my spouse has been affected by my chronic pain?

15. What are three examples of how my chronic pain has affected each of my children? (List each name and give specific examples.)

16. What are three examples each of how chronic pain has affected my mother and father?

17. What are three examples each of how chronic pain has affected my brothers and sisters?

18. What are three examples each of how my chronic pain has affected one or more of my friends?

19. What is the general effect of my chronic pain on my relationships with family and friends? Briefly sum up.

III. Powerlessness

A. What does the word "powerlessness" mean to me?

B. How do I perceive myself as being powerless over chronic pain?

C. Do I feel powerless over drugs? Do I have an alcohol problem?

D. Progression— Has my chronic pain become progressively worse?

1. Do I take ever larger quantities of medication for my pain?

2. Do I combine alcohol with medication?

3. Do I sometimes find I get in trouble because of alcohol and medication combinations?

4. Do I find myself concerned more and more about drug use?

5. Has my physician or any family member expressed concern over my use of medication and/or alcohol?

6. What are three examples of how my chronic pain problem has progressed and led to trouble?

E. Have I made an effort to get my pain problem under control and failed?

1. Have I tried to cut down on medication?

2. Have I attempted to stop all drugs and/or alcohol?

3. Have I switched alcoholic beverages in order to seek better control?

4. Have I set specific time restraints on my drinking?

5. What are five examples of how I have attempted to get control of my chronic pain in the past?

F. Preoccupation— Does life revolve around my pain problem?

1. Does pain regulate my daily activities?

2. Do I sometimes find myself daydreaming excessively about how good it would feel to be free of pain?

3. Do I get angry when other activities prevent people from waiting on me because of my pain?

4. Do I use chronic pain as a trump card in getting my way?

5. Do I use chronic pain to have others do my bidding?

6. What are three examples of my preoccupation with my chronic pain?

G. Avoidance and protection— What do I do so others will not know the true nature of my problem?

1. Have I hidden alcoholic beverages?

2. Have I ever hidden a narcotic, analgesic, or any other mind-altering drug?

3. Am I ashamed about the amount of medication I take?

4. Am I defensive about the narcotics I take?

5. Do I take tranquilizers or sleeping pills? How long? Why?

6. Do I take more medication than my doctor advises me?

7. Do I sneak drinks or drugs?

8. Do I avoid any reference to the use of my drugs?

9. Do I find myself using breath mints or sprays?

10. Do I minimize the amount of drugs I take or the alcohol I consume?

11. Do I avoid people who might find out about my use of drugs?

12. What are five examples of how I have attempted to keep others from finding out about my use of drugs and or alcohol?

H. Loss of control— Do I feel unable to control my life because of chronic pain?

1. How many times have I tried to gain control of my chronic pain problem and failed?

2. How many "cures" have I sought trying to solve my pain problem, only to have my hopes dashed?

3. How many times have I compromised my values because of the pain problem?

4. How many times have I attempted to get off drugs?

5. Have I ever thought of forging prescriptions in order to get drugs?

6. Have I ever purchased drugs on the street?

7. Have I ever had a DUI or been arrested for attempting to get drugs illicitly?

8. What are five examples of how I am losing control of my life because of pain problems?

I. Destructive or dangerous behavior— Have I ever engaged in dangerous behavior because of my chronic pain?

1. Have I ever driven a car under the influence of alcohol or other mind-altering substances (Cocaine, Demerol, Marijuana, Dilaudid, Percoden, Darvon, etc.)?

2. Have I been verbally or physically abusive when under the influence of any drug?

3. Have I ever been advised by a physician to "cut down" or "cut out" medication? How do I react?

4. Have I ever been advised by a physician to "cut down" or not drink at all?

5. What are three examples of how my chronic pain has led to destructive behavior?

J. Shifting responsibility— Do I shift, or try to shift, responsibility for my actions?

1. Do I use chronic pain to justify my actions about which I would ordinarily be ashamed?

2. Do I frequently blame situations and people in order to justify my actions?

3. Do I find myself saying "I'm a nervous wreck!" "I'm tired." "I'm overworked." "It's the pressure."

4. Do I justify taking drugs by saying "If you had my pain, you'd take them too." "Everybody in pain takes drugs." "It's nobody's business what I do!"

5. What are five examples of how I have not accepted responsibility for my actions in dealing with my chronic pain?

K. Difference in perception— Do I see things differently from others?

1. Are others beginning to tell me I have performed some action I can't recall?

2. Do I perceive that action very differently?

3. Have I been told I was intoxicated, but I perceived myself as being totally in control at the time?

4. Have I ever been accused of taking an excessive amount of drugs based on my actions? Have I wondered what tipped the accusers off, since I perceived I acted perfectly natural?

5. Have family, friends, or employers ever shared their concern with me over my drug use?

6. What are three examples of how I have been confronted in the past by my conduct over excessive use of drugs?

L. Review the original responses to these questions on powerlessness. How accurate were your original answers?

M. List eight of the most significant responses which pertain to your being powerless over your chronic pain problem.

Most men and women will benefit greatly by presenting a written First Step to a group, preferably to a Chronic Pain Anonymous gathering. The First Step is a soul-searching, all-out effort to face the truth and shed defenses. A "take no prisoners" type of experience will hopefully represent a new beginning. A superficial effort will likely lead to failure—in a sense, it means an inability to clear the first hurdle in a long race. An excellent First Step is extremely arduous, but the rewards are immense.

## ▲ STEP 2

Came to believe there is a Power greater than ourselves that could restore us to sanity.

### Suggestions Not Commands

Please note that Step 2 issues no command. The Twelve Steps of Alcoholics Anonymous (AA) are not official orders. They are suggestions—very strong suggestions—but suggestions nonetheless. They were put together in the 1930s by troubled people who met together and came up with a philosophy and a set of principles that made sense and worked for them. They were not brilliant philosophers, scientists, academicians, statesmen, or clergymen. They were just ordinary people faced with a lethal problem, people who were simply "sick and tired of being sick and tired." They came up with a formula that has saved them and millions of others since.

### God

Step 2 is an important part of that successful formula. Lots of people run like hell when God is mentioned. "Running like hell" from God is an interesting concept in itself. People who suffer from chronic pain tend to distance themselves from God. Egocentricity is sometimes a big factor. Regardless of the reason, they certainly find themselves on the outside looking in. It's fairly easy for you to be good, grateful, thankful, friendly, outgoing, magnanimous, or cheerful when everything is coming up roses; when you're experiencing pain all day, things aren't coming up roses. When your proximity to God is lost, you must ask the question, "Who moved?" It's easy for a PWCP to move because chronic pain is such a bitter pill to swallow. Often the blame is projected heavenward.

## Power Outside Themselves

One of the major setbacks early AA members had to overcome was that some of them didn't believe in God. To a man and woman, they recognized the need for a spiritual basis, but they had diverse religious affiliations, and there were atheists and agnostics who had to be appeased. They had a problem. They solved it with the "power greater than ourselves concept." If people wished to accept an alternative to "God," as they recognized "God," they simply chose a "power outside themselves." That power might be a group, many groups, another person, a special concept, a telephone pole—whatever or whomever. They just accepted the fact there is a power outside themselves that would restore their sanity.

There's a potential problem here. If a PWCP doesn't accept "God" as his or her Higher Power, it's possible for them to choose some fantastic, guru-type physician, surgeon, psychologist, psychiatrist, or "voodoo practitioner" as the Higher Power. People are people, regardless of their credentials and abilities. Human nature being what it is often sets the stage for bitter disappointment for the PWCP when they put too much faith or trust in another human being (particularly one they're praying will stop their pain). Few people or institutions are perfect. If a PWCP doesn't accept "God," or some other universal "greater power," he or she may use the group consciousness of a particular CPA or AA meeting—many do, and it's a private, individual decision. No one dictates to a CPA member what their "Higher Power" should be. As long as the principle of a "power greater than ourselves" is adhered to, it seems to work famously (with the caution about putting too much stock in other people and human institutions).

## Turmoil

Many a PWCP throws in the towel at this juncture. Some use it as an excuse because it's so much easier to run than stay in the trench and fight to manage the turmoil of chronic pain by turning it over to a Higher Power. Others, quite honestly, just can't cut it. The more intellectual, the more successful professionally, the more likely this is to happen. Non-church-goers are only too eager to point out that they see friends and neighbors going to church with regularity and then witness them tearing each other apart during the week. They point to them and say, "See what phonies they are! See what religion will do for you!" It affords them a great excuse not to even try.

## Higher Power

The people who wrote the Steps had the wisdom not to buy into any of the controversy of religious affiliations. A Higher Power suited them just fine. Most, obviously, accepted God as their Higher Power and worked their program accordingly. All the ancient civilizations had their deities, too. The Babylonians, Egyptians, Greeks, and Romans had their Higher Powers. The most remote Amazonian tribe worships deities. A Higher Power seems to be an integral part of humankind's makeup. The founders of AA did not reinvent the wheel.

## No Hard Rules

There are no hard and fast rules that must be applied to the Steps. Some people, and PWCPs are not an exception, choose to sidestep the Higher Power concept. You might agree that pain has sorely tried your sanity, but that's as far as you will take Step 2. Is this acceptable? Sure it's acceptable; not terribly reasonable, but acceptable. Can you go back to it? Of course. People go back over the Steps many times. They feel they get more out of it every time they put in time and effort. They learn, relearn, study, argue, define, reevaluate, reassess, regress, progress, mull, and change every time they go through each Step. The Steps are dynamic, and the people who take them and work them tend to be dynamic, too.

## Vulnerability

People in pain aren't famous for patience or equanimity. With acute pain, at least there's a light at the end of the tunnel; with chronic pain, much less so. Usually, even with the most stoic person, patience wears thin, tempers are short, love is replaced by hate, and hope is turned into bitterness and despair. Peacefulness and tranquility are destroyed. It's not difficult to imagine how vulnerable someone in chronic pain can be, particularly when such a sensitive issue as your relationship to a Higher Power is questioned and explored. A PWCP tries to keep hostility and anger at bay, but it's relatively easy when your nerves are raw from lack of sleep, constant pain, and lack of understanding and support to go for the throat of another human being when your values are confronted. You can damage and be damaged in a hurry.

## Spirituality

The founders of AA saw a monumental need for spirituality in the program. They recognized a lot of insanity in their midst. They recognized they were fighting a losing battle by themselves. They recognized they had to find something out there to restore their confused and muddled minds. Spirituality means different things to a lot of people. Very simply, it's characterized by an ascendancy of spirit, showing refinement of thought and feeling. Spirituality connotes a good feeling about yourself, a good relationship with your Higher Power, and most important, a special, wonderful relationship with those around you. Spirit is the thinking, motivating, feeling part of any person, consciousness, and thought (as distinguished from the body). Spirituality in AA is the power plant that makes a person run, that gives a person sparkle and life.

## Trust

A PWCP must learn to trust again. Historically, most have much to be distrustful about. They placed their trust in others and, for the most part, that trust didn't prove helpful. Most have run the gauntlet of multiple surgeries with little or no relief. Most have essentially given up hope. Most are hooked on pills. Why should they trust anyone or anything? You have to have courage and tenacity to have suffered all the indignities common to people with chronic pain and still be able to trust once more.

A truly spiritual person *can* renew his or her trust. Spirituality allows you to trust a Higher Power, to trust that Higher Power to give you back your sanity. If you are looking for a miracle, the Higher Power certainly seems to be a logical place to look.

## Spiritual Awareness

Many people who work their AA program talk about a "spiritual awakening" experienced after getting involved with the Steps. Most seem to be almost reticent to talk about it; others want to talk about nothing else. Whether the experience is compared to being struck by lightning or a simple lifting of the intellectual clouds, they all seem to be moved mentally and physically. Whatever it is, the spiritual awakening has a profound effect. If there were just some way it could be framed in time, we would have a happier chronic pain populace, too. It's unfortunate that we can't bottle this awakening. It seems to hit people at different stages of the Steps, but those who have the experience are most certainly changed by it. The AA saying "Bring the body and the mind will follow" takes on new significance. Somewhere, somehow, the lights get turned on and all of the sudden, a lot of things make sense. Many attribute it to their Higher Power. Parenthetically, the spiritual awakening seems to happen to those who just plug away at it; the St. Paul suddenly-struck-by-lightning scenario isn't the rule. Many just seem to be slugging it out, and they have a sublime, marvelous, almost indescribable experience as their reward. If you have suffered for years with pain, you could certainly use such an experience.

## Denial

When it comes to recognizing a Higher Power, you can bet the defense mechanisms come home to roost. Denial is a major factor. "Who needs a Higher Power?" Proud people use denial like a sword. Many refuse to deal with the thought that God has anything to do with them or anything in their lives. They suppress their thoughts. The mere thought of a supreme being "directing traffic" makes them uncomfortable, so they consciously tune out.

## Rationalization

Rationalization runs rampant in dealing with a Higher Power. "If there was a God, He would not allow me to suffer so!"; therefore, there is no God. Since there is no Higher Power in their minds, then there will be no one to answer to. (Now there is a handy bit of rationalization.) Not having to answer for your transgressions definitely lightens your load!

## Delusions

Delusions allow you to continue to ignore all of your problems. "This next surgery will get rid of my pain." "The new high-powered medical whiz from Good Luck, South Dakota, will solve my problem!" These, after five or more unsuccessful surgeries, are classic delusions. Defense mechanisms are a formidable force. They can muddy the waters very quickly when venturing into spirituality.

## Sanity

Chronic Pain Anonymous affords a comfortable climate in which to discuss the concept of Higher Power and the question of restoration to sanity. When sanity is discussed, the defense mechanisms come out in full force. Chronic pain tends to put people out of touch with reality. Psychiatrically, insanity is a term applied to a variety of specialized mental disorders, functional or organic, in which the personality is seriously disorganized. Pain that never leaves can seriously disorganize any personality. It takes infinite time, patience, kindness, wisdom, perspicacity, love, tenderness, and good common sense to deal with people suffering from long-term chronic pain. The majority of all Anonymous members are the first to admit there must be a Higher Power generating their groups or they would have fallen apart long ago. Chronic pain does strange things to your mind. So often the straightening-out process needs all the help available. Getting straight is the easy part; staying straight is the tough part. CPA offers a place for that to happen.

## Trust and Belief

The person suffering from chronic pain is asked to find the trust and belief in an existing Higher Power, outside themselves, that can restore sanity. PWCPs have taken hundreds of risks before, they hurt so much, and most are willing to try anything. If their physicians told them to stand on their heads in the middle of traffic three times a day or burn incense in the bathroom, many would not hesitate. Step 2 simply asks you to try something new and different. It asks the PWCP to take a chance, and make a real effort to believe in a source of untapped power that can unscramble your mind so you can think logically again. Finite beings do not solve your problems. Material things like drugs just make everything worse. Now PWCPs are asked to up the ante and put their trust and belief in an infinite power that can help fix them. The Higher Power does not ask for a person's insurance policy number before tackling the job. The financial price is absolutely nothing—the real price is the abandonment of pride and a real shift of responsibility to yourself. No one can do it for you. You and the person in pain must do it, and it must come from the heart.

### Pride

To admit that your mind is less than perfect is most difficult if you're ruled by pride. Step 1, aptly performed, is designed to demonstrate how badly things really are going. The physical problems are hard to deny or ignore; the mental derangements are easier to project, deny, repress, rationalize, or suppress. Assuming you have done an honest First Step, the chances are you have readily seen how your mind has played an active part in the chronic pain. Tortured bodies are frequently accompanied by tortured minds. The ministrations of human beings have failed to alleviate the pain, so it's time to try another tack. God, or the Higher Power, is up to the task. The PWCP just has to have the faith that it's possible.

## ▲ STEP 3

Made a decision to turn our will and our lives over to the care of God *as we understood Him.*

## Action

Step 3 is show time. It's time for action. The rumination is over. The philosophizing is history. A conscious decision has to be made to "turn our will and our lives over" to God, a Higher Power. That's quite a task!

Actually, talking about "turning our will and our lives over" is fairly easy. People talk non-stop about it. Perhaps they feel if they keep talking loud and hard enough, they'll even convince themselves they really mean it. Mental "lightweights" spend about two minutes thinking about this Step. They do it quickly and it means absolutely nothing to them. But, for the great majority, this Step is profound.

## Turn it Over!

People in the program tend to bicker constantly about which Step is the most important. There probably is no answer because one is predicated on another. Many like to think Step 3 outstrips the others because it's dynamic: you must do it every day of your life. All of us have hurdles to clear daily. Everyday obstacles are thrown in front of us, crises occur, we get dumped and stepped on, nothing seems to go right, and this Step suggests "Turn it over!"

Do you think that this is easy to do? Do you think that turning over excruciating pain, and probably an obsession with drugs, is easy? A person suffering with pain day and night doesn't want to be told to just "turn it over!" He or she wants the pain to stop 100%. They want it to go away. When "turning it over" comes up, PWCPs tend to become graphic as to where and what we can do with the advice. They're only interested in something to make the terrible hurt stop. Every time they cough, sneeze, have a bowel movement, or twist the wrong way, they feel a thousand volts go screaming down the back of their legs. Having air flow over their arm from an open car window is enough to bring tears to their eyes. If chronic headache is their problem, their heads feel like the Russian Army just walked through them. "Turning the pain over" doesn't seem like much of a solution to them. They quickly forget, however, that they've probably had the pain for years and if there was a physical solution, it would already have been put into motion.

"Turning it over" doesn't mean there will be an instantaneous cure. It's unlikely you will be able to clear seven feet in the high jump the same day. When an alcoholic or drug addict "turns it over," his or her problems don't stop. Their burden may lighten a bit, but a long road lies ahead. If the message springs from the heart, however, it's a good start.

## Denial and Rationalization

The "decision to turn our will and our lives over" to the care of a Higher Power provides ample exercise for the defense mechanisms. A little voice inside your head denies such an action could possibly help. "If God cared at all, He would have taken the horrible pain away already!" Denial stops any action, or leads to half measures. If an idea is repugnant or thought to be foolish, you can bet it will be suppressed or buried in the subconscious. Rationalization can be used effectively to do virtually nothing. "If 'turning it over' were an answer, someone surely would have told me about it before. It's a waste of time and effort. It's asking too much from me!" If you're using narcotics, you can depend on rationalization defeating any motivation to turn it over. Turning it over might mean that you must give up the pills. That thought would absolutely terrify anyone addicted to tranquilizers or analgesics. The more supple the mind, the more imaginative the rationalization.

## Strength from Group

That is why CPA or a like group of peers is needed to listen patiently to the hundreds of excuses and effectively confront them kindly and reasonably. Most PWCPs have used the same arguments themselves in the past, so they understand what's really going on. They understand how difficult it is to let go and let God into their lives. For them, the path has been well-traveled.

## Faith

The typical person in chronic pain is fairly worn out when it comes to faith. Usually faith has long gone by the boards. Faith is an unquestioned belief not requiring proof or evidence. The PWCP generally has had his or her fill of disillusionment when it comes to faith. It takes a lot of faith to submit to surgery five or ten times, for instance, and each time make no improvement or end up in worse condition. The surgeon couldn't produce any evidence or proof that the problem would be fixed. It's not possible, yet all kinds of people submit themselves to surgical procedures every day on blind trust. Most of the time, their faith is justified. Not so, however, with chronic pain patients. The PWCP is typically skeptical when asked to trust anyone or anything again. They have been burned too many times. Now they are asked to let God, or a Higher Power, be the surgeon. They are requested to make a conscious decision to "turn their will" over to God. It's indeed a mind-boggling concept.

## Desperation

Will is the power of making a reasonable choice or decision, or controlling your own actions. However,

Step 3 requests that your will and your life be turned over to God or a Higher Power. It means surrendering the power of reasoned choice to someone or something else. How many people have the guts to do such a thing? Few rational people are willing to give up the power of reasoned choice. A person would have to be fairly desperate to do such a thing. A PWCP, though, is usually desperate enough. An alcoholic or drug addict is desperate enough. When you see life going down the tubes, they're desperate enough. When an anorexic or bulemic patient has to be supported with intravenous feeding or die, he or she is desperate enough. When the compulsive gambler or sex addict witnesses life disintegrating, he or she is desperate enough.

## Heart

If belief doesn't come from the heart, the PWCP isn't going to make it. That belief has to be unquestioned. Faith must be like steel. It must be unwavering. If belief is halfhearted or superficial, then Step 3 will be a waste of time. Where do you find unquestioned belief? How can you be assured your belief is strong enough? How do you know the Higher Power has enough horsepower to take the pain away? How do you know He is even interested? How do you know there's a Higher Power? PWCPs are being asked to come up with unshakable trust and faith in a Higher Power and turn their will, the power of choice—essentially their most valuable possession—over to Him or Her, a Supreme Being, as He or She is understood.

## Courage

It takes a terrific amount of faith to turn over all of your worldly goods to another mortal. You have to trust another to the hilt to do such a thing. Worldly goods are hard to come by. You might turn over some of your worldly goods, but the chances are fairly good you'd pick and choose, and most wouldn't do it at all. "Let the suckers do it!" would probably be the normal response. Assuming you had the courage to do it, it would be an act of the highest confidence. There are some churches that function somewhat in that manner. We have witnessed or read about some of the less elevating consequences. We know of religious orders where men and women leave all their worldly possessions at the door when they enter a religious order and, of course, that takes a great deal of courage.

Essentially, the person suffering from chronic pain is asked to go a step further. He or she is asked to hand over will, the ability to make a reasoned choice. The will is much more valuable than any material asset they own. It's a quantum leap and, understandably, many PWCPs hesitate to jump. If you fully realize the implications, the hesitation is well-founded.

## Higher Power

The other part of Step 3's equation is the Higher Power. You can talk to a human being, look up his or her Dun and Bradstreet rating, and investigate their personal background—things you can hang your hat on. But turning over your will and life to something or someone so nebulous and mystical as a Higher Power demands a large chunk of faith. "In God We Trust" is not just a phrase on the back of a coin. If you think about it, however, you really do place your trust and faith in finite beings in hundreds of ways every day . We trust that the driver bearing down on us from the opposite side of the road isn't going to hit us head-on. We trust that the airline pilot knows what he or she is doing. We trust the lawyer who represents us in court. We trust physicians in their capacity.

Those people are *nothing* next to a Higher Power. God, as we understand Him, is responsible for our next heartbeat, our next breath. If we can accept that, we can certainly accept the fact that God as we understand Him can fix anyone, whenever He pleases! Step 3 doesn't say the "fixing" will happen. It seems unlikely that demanding to be fixed would get us very far. Making a decision to turn it over sets up no demands. The PWCP is just putting a foot in the door, exposing the self to a magnificent presence, and saying he or she is willing to make a commitment.

## Turning it Over

Step 3 is dynamic because people learn to do it all day, every day. They develop a powerful belief that what they can't handle, God can. They constantly embrace a silent prayer, the Serenity Prayer:

*God grant me the serenity to accept the things I cannot change,*

*the courage to change the things I can,*

*and the wisdom to know the difference.*

Every frustration, every sharp visceral pain, every injustice, and every lousy break gets handed over. God, or a Higher Power, has "broad shoulders." When running into something greatly disturbing, PWCPs accept the fact they can't change it, and they can hand it over. If they can put a dent in it, they take a whack at it. It's hoped God will give them the wisdom to know the difference between can and cannot, and what a beautiful philosophy of life! It's not difficult to see how such a philosophy would significantly change a person with chronic pain. Several years of frustration does not do much for your attitude or personality. The best of the best tend to give up all hope, then depression follows. Hopelessness and helplessness become constant companions, affecting everyone around them. It's hard to be the life of the party when being eaten alive by pain. Adoption of this new philosophy of life is no guarantee of being pain-free either, but "by God" it's the positive new start PWCPs need. It takes a good man or woman to give it 100%. Half measures won't succeed. "Any length" should become part of your vocabulary. You will need constant support. You will need to be reminded vigorously and often. You will need to discover prayer again. And yes, indeed, you will need to be prepared for big changes in your life.

## ▲ STEP 4

Made a searching and fearless moral inventory of ourselves.

### Time

Opinion is divided as to when Step 4 should be done. Some claim it should be completed within the first month or so after you begin the CPA program; others like to see people take their time. There are really no set rules. All agree that it should be thorough. Since thoroughness usually means an investment of sufficient time, perhaps there is wisdom in taking several months to complete the personal inventory this Step requires.

### Serious Business

People in constant pain are not usually patient. True to form, alcoholics and other addicts win no prizes for patience, either. A good moral inventory smacks more of the cool, calculating accountant—careful, exact, and unremitting. There's little or no room for flippancy. Chronic pain is a deadly business; Step 4 is also a serious business.

## Fearless Inventory

The purpose of Step 4 is not to point fingers, flail around, or make yourself miserable by recounting past sins. Moralistic flagellation has no place here. This isn't an exercise in dealing out punishment. People with chronic pain don't need to be beaten up any more, mentally or physically. What they do need is an honest, searching, and fearless inventory, a good straightforward, cold-blooded assessment of what has transpired in their lives and what's going on now. They need to delve into anything that might get in the way of getting well. Few people are perfect, and everyone needs to take out the mental garbage periodically.

## Getting On With It

A conscientious inventory will probably dredge up some guilt, fear, frustration, depression, anxiety, and a host of uncomfortable feelings for you. So be it. Step 4 can't be taken without receiving some lumps, but that's not its purpose. When taking a critical look at your weaknesses, it's unlikely that elation follows. It's a job most people avoid as long as possible. Procrastination is only human, but taking an inventory is such an important part of working your program that foot-dragging must be thwarted. Getting on with it and getting it done must be the priority. Everything is hard if you suffer with chronic pain—nothing comes easy. The Fourth Step is a lot of mental and physical work and it means a significant investment of time. A defeated, weak, vacillating, and irresolute person will not even try. A person who is fed up with being sick will try doing his or her best with the inventory, letting the chips fall where they may.

## In-Depth Approach

Needless to say, this Step should be written out, just as the First Step was. Actually, a good First makes an easier Fourth. Much of the same information will surface. The Fourth, however, is a much more in-depth search. The First was an all-out effort to explore just how your life has become mucked up through constant, unremitting pain. If an honest effort was expended and you find that, indeed, pain hasn't fouled up your life, the CPA program ended before it really got started. Why fix something if it's not broken? But if the reverse is true, then headway has already been made on the Fourth Step. Much of the same territory will be probed again, but this time in a more thorough and fearless fashion.

## Let It All Hang Out!

Fear is a feeling of anxiety and agitation caused by the presence of danger, evil, or pain. It implies uneasiness, apprehension, dread, and terror. A fearless moral inventory connotes the opposite. The inventory process is attacked vigorously without any uneasiness, apprehension, or terror. "Let it all hang out" isn't a bad attitude. The PWCP, probably for the first time in years, says "Oh, the hell with it!" and plunges ahead with the task. Chronic pain wears you down and negativity may pervade the very fiber of your existence. Negativity, however, has no place in Step 4. It needs to be downgraded and put aside.

## Guidance and Direction

The following material provides the groundwork for a solid Fourth Step. Obviously, you don't have to use the suggested inventory form or any part of it. It does seem to help, however, from both the searching and fearless perspectives, in that it forces you to look under some ugly rocks that probably would have been ignored. It's difficult to use this format (if done honestly) and not do a thorough inventory. Most PWCPs need some guidance and direction, and this format has been designed to make the task easier and more user-friendly.

## Sponsor

CPA is designed specifically for people suffering from chronic pain. New members need to seek out and ask older experienced members for help. Sponsorship is an extremely important, necessary function for all Anonymous groups. When launching into Step 4, a sponsor can provide priceless assistance. Having been over the road themselves, sponsors usually are able to steer you around potential pitfalls and help you maintain balance and perspective. When doing the Fourth, the newcomer will need encouragement and a special kind of gentle prodding. A good sponsor will fill the bill admirably and almost guarantee a successful Step.

## Writing It Out

Writing out the Fourth Step helps immensely. If it helped doing the First Step, it will help even more now for all the same reasons: crystallizing thought, provoking investigative thinking, slowing down the process, and many other good reasons. Again, a sponsor can help keep you from beating yourself up mentally, keep you focused, and may even help with the prose. When you begin to examine your dark side, it helps to have a good pilot to lean on. Ultimately, there's nothing better to lean on than God or your Higher Power. God is a good listener. Prayer is merely conversation with God. It makes sense when doing the Fourth to get God on the line.

My priest friend tells me people are always asking him to pray for them. His standard reply is, "Say hello

to the Boss yourself! He'll be glad to hear from you."
There's much wisdom in such advice.

## Fourth Step Inventory

### Fear

1. Am I afraid of being rejected?
2. Am I afraid to speak in a group for fear of letting people know how little I know? Am I afraid of being made fun of?
3. Is my pain an excuse not to go out in public?
4. Am I afraid of groups?
5. Am I afraid I will fail at this program, like at everything else?
6. Am I afraid to allow others to get to know me, because they will know how I really am?
7. Am I afraid of accepting the responsibility of getting well? Do I wish to do the work necessary to get well?
8. Am I afraid of facing the world without drugs?
9. Am I afraid of going back to work?
10. Am I afraid I can't function well in the work world?
11. Am I ashamed of my physical appearance?
12. Am I afraid of competition?
13. Am I afraid of sharing my feelings with others?
14. What are three outstanding examples of how my fear might interfere with my recovery?

### Resentment

1. Do I feel like a parasite in the family unit, living off others?
2. Do I feel frustrated having to depend on others to take care of me, provide my meals, and do my laundry?
3. Do I carry my own weight?
4. Do I hate my own complaining?
5. Do I resent the health of my family and friends?

6. Do I resent having to wait for others to serve my needs?

7. Do I resent not being asked to do things of which I am capable?

8. Do people treat me as inferior because of my pain problem?

9. Do I resent the way I have to beg for pills?

10. Do people think I abuse drugs? Does it make me angry?

11. Do I resent the way drugs were prescribed for me?

12. Do I resent the money I have spent on my pain problem, and my present financial state as a result?

13. What are three examples of how my resentment might interfere with my recovery?

**Alibis**

1. Do I use my pain problem to get out of work?

2. Do I use my pain to avoid things I do not enjoy—parties, social engagements, church, etc.?

3. Am I physically able to do more work than I do?

4. Do I exaggerate ailments in order to get drugs?

5. Do I find myself inventing reasons to get more medications?

6. Do I find myself justifying uncalled-for conduct by blaming it on my pain?

7. Do I use partial truth and embellish it?

8. Have I abandoned many projects because of my pain?

9. Do I hide behind my pain problem, using it as an excuse to withdraw from things I do not care to discuss?

10. Do I use chronic pain as an excuse for not functioning well as a mother, father, sister, brother, etc.?

11. Do I use chronic pain as an excuse not to keep up my physical attractiveness?

12. Do I use chronic pain as an excuse not to honor my marital conjugal rights?

13. Have I used my pain problem as an excuse to allow myself to put on weight?

14. Have I used my pain problem as an excuse not to exercise?

15. Have I used my pain problem as an excuse to gain attention and pity?

16. What are three examples of how my use of alibis might interfere with my recovery?

**Pride**

1. Do I no longer care how I look?

2. Do I read good books and try to keep my mind occupied with constructive ideas and interesting thoughts?

3. Has chronic pain led me to lose my self-respect?

4. Am I too proud to share my true feelings with others?

5. Has chronic pain led me to lie about how things really are in my home, work, and social life?

6. Has my pride kept me from looking at my behavior as it really is?

7. Do I sometimes become grandiose in my ideas in order not to face the facts?

8. Am I ready to admit to any weakness on my part?

9. Do I look to certain people who I know will support me in my thinking?

10. Do I put up a false front in public?

11. Do I use chronic pain to cover my own inadequacies?

12. Am I too proud to admit I am hooked on drugs?

13. Am I too proud to associate myself with self-help programs?

14. Do I consider myself as being superior and a special circumstance?

15. Do I consider myself better than most people with chronic pain?

16. What are three examples of how pride might interfere with my recovery?

**Greed**

1. Do I want to be center stage most of the time? Do I use chronic pain sometimes to that end?

2. Do I ever use chronic pain to get my way?

3. Do I hoard pills and save some for special occasions?

4. Do I want more service from my family because I feel I earn it with my suffering?

5. Do I use chronic pain as a mechanism to get money from the state, insurance company, etc.?

6. Am I honest? Do I try to embellish my pain for financial gain?

7. Do I feel I do not get the proper respect from my family and friends because of my predicament?

8. Am I aggressive? Am I assertive to the point where I must get my way even if it hurts others?

9. Do I usually think first about my needs and second about the needs of others?

10. Have immediate friends or family alluded to my being spoiled or pampered because of my pain?

11. Do I thoroughly enjoy telling my pain story in public?

12. What are three good examples in my life and experience of how greed might interfere with my recovery?

**Anger**

1. Do I anger easily? Do I use anger to get my own way?

2. Does it make me mad I can't convey to people how much I suffer?

3. Do I ever have tantrums? Do I use them to take advantage of my family and friends?

4. Do I blow things out of proportion, and use little things to get others off an uncomfortable subject?

5. Do I blame chronic pain for my loss of control?

6. Do I think my pain tends to get worse when I get angry?

7. Do I use more painkilling drugs after an emotional flare-up?

8. Do I deliberately provoke anger in others, then sit back and watch the fight?

9. How angry am I now, compared to when I did not have chronic pain?

10. Do I internalize my anger? Do I ever level with my family and friends about the things that anger me?

11. Am I physically violent? Do I immediately apologize and then wonder why things do not revert to the way they were?

12. Are people afraid of my anger? Have they told me so? Do I use my anger as a weapon?

13. Am I angry with God because of my pain?

14. Am I angry with myself?

15. Am I angry about the breaks I have had in life, the pain I have, and the way my family treats me?

16. Do I feel my anger is justified?

17. Does my anger cause me abdominal pain?

18. Do I think self-hatred has anything to do with my lashing out at people?

19. What are three personal examples of how my anger might interfere with my recovery?

**Envy**

1. Do I envy people because they don't have chronic pain and I do?

2. Do I envy the way so-called "normal" people can exercise and I can't?

3. Do I envy others the material goods chronic pain has blocked me from gaining?

4. Do I envy the freedom everyone else has to get around and do things, while I'm largely restricted in activities?

5. Do I envy my friends their physical attributes?

6. Do I envy the way others are socially acceptable and I'm not? Does chronic pain keep me indoors?

7. Has chronic pain turned me into a cynic? Do I criticize others to make myself look better?

8. Do I put others down to make myself look better?

9. Am I bitter over the progress others, whom I consider inferior, have made?

10. Do I wish other people had my pain?

11. Do I envy my partner in his or her freedom and my lack of it?

12. Do I blame my lack of money on chronic pain?

13. Is my envy such that I find myself hating others?

14. Do I spend much of my time spinning wistful and unrealistic dreams?

15. Have people accused me of envy?

16. What are three examples of how envy has affected my life and how it might interfere with my recovery?

**Humility**

1. Do I truly recognize weakness in myself?

2. Do I have the humility to accept myself as an addict?

3. Do I catch myself voicing self-deprecation, hoping others will argue against me?

4. Am I truly powerless over chronic pain?

5. Do I think I can manage my pain problem by myself, without help?

6. Do I have the humility to accept the fact I am powerless over mind-altering drugs?

7. Am I ready to take advice instead of give it?

8. Am I inclined to think of myself as "soaring with eagles," and other PWCPs as "turkeys?"

9. Do I think I'm one notch above the average person with chronic pain?

10. Do I despise weakness in others?

11. Do I look upon myself as being able to tolerate more pain than most?

12. Do I really think that my family and friends are largely responsible for my problem?

13. Do I dislike going to CPA meetings when others are going out to have a good time?

14. Am I ashamed to associate with other PWCPs?

15. Do I look down on alcoholics, heroin addicts, and cocaine addicts?

16. What are three examples of how my lack of humility might interfere with my recovery?

**Patience**

1. Do I seem to want everything yesterday?

2. Have I lost patience with my physician before really giving him or her an adequate chance?

3. Have I lost patience with God?

4. Have I lost patience with my partner or family?

5. Do I use chronic pain to excuse myself when I become aggressive for inappropriate reasons?

6. Am I getting short-tempered lately, as compared with six months ago?

7. Am I ashamed of the way I fly into a rage?

8. Have I lost friends because of being impatient?

9. Am I more patient with myself than others?

10. Have I set timetables and expect everyone else to comply? Are they reasonable?

11. Do I become disturbed when my plans do not turn out as quickly as I had hoped?

12. Do I wait until my painkiller is due, or do I lose patience and take it before the appointed time?

13. Have family and/or friends pointed out my lack of patience?

14. Have I pushed for surgery because of my lack of patience?

15. Do I have a tendency to expect immediate relief from pain?

16. What are three examples of how impatience might interfere with my recovery?

**Guilt**

1. Do I make people around me feel guilty because of their lack of attention to my needs?

2. Do I think God is punishing me for my sins by inflicting pain on me?

3. Do I feel guilty about the time my family must take to meet my needs?

4. Do I feel guilty about all the money spent on my pain problem?

5. Do people accuse me of whining?

6. Do I enjoy comparing my complaints with others? Do I frequently get into "Can you top this?" pain contests?

7. Do I wallow in my guilt? Has anyone ever suggested that I do?

8. Do I have a tendency to punish those around me when I am in pain, then offer a superficial apology?

9. Have I made people who are taking care of me cry? How do I feel about it?

10. Do I put myself down, feigning false humility?

11. Do I go to great lengths describing my pain to those around me, provoking guilt in them?

12. Do I hope people will feel sorry for me? Do I promote such a feeling in others?

13. Do I sometimes think I invest a lot of energy in trying to make people as miserable as I am?

14. Do I feel guilty about my weight?

15. Do I feel guilty about my lack of exercise?

16. What are three specific examples of how guilt might interfere with my recovery?

**Forgiveness**

1. Am I presently harboring a grudge against my partner, children, or any friends?

2. Do I hate slim, active, and healthy-looking people?

3. Do I seek out equally miserable people for company?

4. Have I been accused of talking too much and listening too little?

5. Have I been accused of little understanding?

6. Do I find myself dwelling on uncomfortable past events?

7. Do I find my hate grows with time?

8. Do I forgive God for my pain?

9. Have I recently asked God for forgiveness of uncharitable thoughts or actions?

10. Has anyone accused me of meanness lately?

11. Do I enjoy my hate?

12. Do I like unforgiving people?

13. Do I heap blame on others, like family, friends, and physicians?

14. Am I generally a "down with people" person?

15. What are three examples of how my unforgiving nature might interfere with my recovery?

**Sloth**

1. Do people tell me I am lazy?

2. Do I loathe exercise?

3. Would I rather moan and groan about my pain than work hard physically trying to change?

4. Is the word "can't" a major part of my language?

5. Do I think I am aggressive in trying to get well, or have I just given up and allowed others to assume responsibility for me?

6. Do I put a sub-minimal effort in following the instructions of my physical therapists?

7. Do I try to walk farther and faster every day?
8. What are three examples of how my sloth might interfere with my recovery?

It makes sense to assemble all the written materials after completing Step 4 and read it over several times. Usually, as in most inventories, there are both assets and liabilities to be counted. In chronic pain it's easy to find yourself wallowing in negativity and sometimes self-pity. If you're not careful, it's easy to dwell on the melancholy side of the inventory. Once more, a good sponsor can help prevent this from happening. It helps to count your assets, too.

A PWCP often has not had much success to brag, extol, or generally just feel good about. Doing a good Fourth Step usually results in more than just a breath of fresh air. It results in a sense of real accomplishment. Every new bit of success provides a small kick of adrenaline. Someone suffering from chronic pain appreciates any boost. Some claim the boost is not so little. Regardless, the climb up the ladder progresses.

## ▲ STEP 5

Admitted to God, to ourselves, and to another human being the exact nature of our wrongs.

### Presentation

Step 4 demands considerable time and effort, perhaps weeks to months, if done properly. Not so with Step 5. The Fifth Step is more about humility and action. Momentum shouldn't be lost. You should move along to the Fifth quickly. Too often people drag their feet, particularly people laden with pride. They discovered getting it together in the Fourth Step was no picnic, but presenting it is a different story.

## Humility and Pride

Humility does not come easily to proud people. They can admit things to God and to themselves, but when it comes to other human beings, they get cold feet. They find that about as easy as running a four-minute mile. When it comes time for a proud person to relate distressing and humiliating memories dredged from the murky recesses of the mind, it's not only difficult to do, it's sometimes nearly impossible. Every admission chokes. It's hard to let go. The proud person holds on to deep secrets, and some even die with them. But the proud person doesn't get well.

## Sweeping Out the Mental Attic

"As sick as your secrets" is a saying underpinned by a lot of truth. The defense mechanisms, particularly suppression and repression, keep you mentally sick. Your mental attic needs to be swept out and you can't do a half-hearted job and expect success. A thorough mental housecleaning entails admissions to another human being. It doesn't entail a cursory, offhanded, flippant admission. The Fifth Step asks for admission of the "exact nature of our wrongs." The more honest, humble and exact, the more likely the success. Mental health plays a large part in anyone's physical health. A person agonizing in chronic pain needs all the mental health he or she can muster. Detailing the mental garbage, the transgressions, and the secrets accumulated over time is done in Step 5.

## Value

Psychologists and psychiatrists are the first in line to verify the value of mental housecleaning. Some people spend a small fortune going through this process with psychologists and psychiatrists over a period of years. Confession has been an integral part of the Catholic Church forever. The priest represents God. The penitent confesses to God, but a mortal pronounces absolution; the priest is the middleman. The psychological benefits of the confessional are unquestioned. Most people with a religious bent have little trouble accepting the concept of the Fifth Step.

## Isolation

Isolation is a critical problem typified in chronic pain. In time, people tend to cut themselves off from family, friends and yes, also from God or a Higher Power. They withdraw into their own little worlds and build barriers. They will not let anyone in, and they will not come out.

## Self-Pity

Self-pity feeds on itself. CPA forces you out of isolation, but part of that process is the Fifth Step. You must vacate the stronghold when you do the Fifth. You must venture forth and bare your soul. You must reach out to an infinite source, but also to another finite being. You can't do that from an isolated position. A major breach in the wall of isolation is required.

## Depression

People who isolate themselves tend to be depressed. They find themselves in deep mental holes; they need to climb out, but it's easier said than done. The Fifth helps them out of their holes, but the beautiful thing is they do it largely by themselves. They can take the credit, taking a bow for a change. A neurochemical didn't lift the depression. It's small wonder why PWCPs feel so good about the program and themselves. God helped, a sponsor might have helped, CPA offered support, but when it came down to it, the PWCP squared his or her shoulders and did the Step. In doing so, significant progress was made by stepping from mental darkness into sunlight. When things are cold and damp, sunlight feels pretty good. An excellent Fifth Step contributes greatly to standing tall, with straight shoulders and chin held high.

## Another Human Being

A major obstacle in the Fifth Step is "admitted to another human being." A common response is, "Do I *really* have to use another human being?" The answer is yes. Sitting down with another human being takes the guesswork out of it. It brings it from a supernatural level to a natural level. It cuts out "maybe" and "perhaps" and faces practical reality. When your wrongs are presented to another human being, you tend to become more concrete and honest. It's easy to con yourself, but more difficult to con another human being, particularly if they've been in your shoes—it's hard to con a con. Obviously, the "other" human being must be chosen with care. It helps to locate someone with Fifth Step experience. A sponsor might be good or bad. The clergy is a good resource, but it's helpful to have someone who understands the Twelve Step program, preferably someone who is in the program. Sometimes a qualified person who is a complete stranger fills the bill admirably. The "other" must be a sensitive and caring person, but they will not offer absolution. Forgiveness only comes from within you.

## No Rules

Interestingly enough, some CPA members go through this Step gradually, taking it by degrees. Some even use several "others" to complete it. Some save the really onerous material for a special person and the simple things for another. The founding members of the Twelve Step movement didn't seem to go for hard and fast rules. They were apparently more interested in a simple, basic, honest, heartfelt, sincere, genuine, and exact disclosure of what emerged from the Fourth Step. "Keeping it simple" seems to be a major key to success in the program.

### Solo Exercise

The other human being doesn't act as a judge or jury in the Fifth Step. Neither is there an absolution or a sentence. You will not get a fifteen-yard penalty or life imprisonment. Certainly the other human being may offer advice and counsel on the quality of information you present. If your performance is superficial, hasty, nebulous, phony, or obsequious, you will be informed so without much ceremony. All in all, the Fifth Step is an individual or solo exercise and its success will depend on your honesty and sincerity.

### Response

After Step 5, people usually feel great relief. One thousand pounds has been lifted from very tired shoulders. In chronic pain, it's easy to feel helpless. Physical pain may cause people to grind their teeth and lose their breath or even scream when it hits, but the mind can positively influence how the PWCP responds.

A good Fifth Step also solidifies your position as a member of CPA. It signifies that you are working your program. Frequently, it's not a one-time perfor-mance. You may do it several times. In the fellowship of CPA, it sends a message to your "pain pals" that you are trying. Completing the Fifth evokes a mark of respect from fellow members, whether vocalized or not. Others went through it, and they know how hard it was and the relief they enjoyed when it was successfully completed. People outside the program don't fully realize what's entailed. Men and women in CPA know what the Fifth Step is all about. Men and women in all Anonymous organizations understand because they've been down the same road, too. Most Twelve Step members look at the Fifth Step as a real landmark in their recovery.

## ▲ STEP 6

Were entirely ready to have God remove all these defects of character.

### Character Defects

Step 4 took care of the discovery of your shortcomings, and Step 5 the admission. Now, for Step 6, you must be prepared to abandon the defects of character. It's one thing to admit transgressions and their accompanying character defects; it's another to prepare to jettison them.

### Change

When you've been acting a certain way for years, change doesn't come easily. Through the inventory process, some PWCPs might have discovered they were using pain to gain personal advantage. With chronic pain, some become adept at manipulating those around them. They exploit their condition by using pain to get what they want. They learn to manipulate their partner, friends, and family. It happens. The significant others surrounding the PWCP might find themselves taking on the role of codependents, which makes them just as sick or sicker than the one with the pain. This, of course, is a rather glaring character defect for all concerned.

## Preparing to "Let Go"

Step 6 states: If there are character defects, and we know it, we must be ready to have God remove them. To some this represents a major life change. Those willing to let God remove their character defects must be prepared to let go. Some are unwilling to pay that price. One faction wants to make their pain the responsibility of others; the ones who are willing to change, however, take on the responsibility themselves. They stand ready and willing for God to remove their character defects. They stand ready for change.

## Obsession

Alcoholics become obsessed with alcohol. Heroin addicts become obsessive about heroin. Cocaine addicts are obsessed with cocaine. Sex addicts are obsessed with sex. Gamblers are obsessive about gambling. PWCPs become obsessed with their pain. When alcoholics become preoccupied with alcohol, they think about booze constantly and life revolves around alcohol. They can't imagine socializing without a drink in hand. Life without alcohol doesn't seem worth it. They know it's killing them and destroying their home, work and social life, yet they continue to drink. The same obsession is true of all addictions—life revolves around the addiction.

In chronic pain, life revolves around the pain. Every waking action seems to be affected by it. Pain becomes an abnormal preoccupation and one difficult to alter. You can't sleep, eat, walk, talk, sit, cry, or laugh without experiencing some backlash of pain. No rational person wants the pain; they welcome any small relief. As time goes on, they find the obsession is such that the pain governs their lives. They don't control it; it controls them.

## Drug Dependency

A relatively common finding among PWCPs is a dependency on drugs. "Dependency" is another word for "addiction." For a PWCP, that spells double trouble. Dependency on codeine, percodan, dilaudid, demoral, morphine, methadone, marijuana, alcohol, tranquilizers, and sleeping pills is common; a large percent of PWCPs end up dependent on drugs. It's absolutely scary.

In chronic pain, the obsession has to go. You must stand ready to remove all your defects of character; obsession is an Olympic-size defect. Drug addiction, of course, is an obsession culminating in abstinence or in death. The combination of chronic pain and drug addiction is a formidable foe, one that demands an "any lengths" approach, an all-out war. Only the best survive the struggle.

Hundreds of thousands of people have taken the Sixth Step and are healthy, successful human beings today. They came to AA, hat in hand, stating that they were ready to give up their character defects, and they did it in a state of high anxiety, hoping and praying their obsessions and other character defects would be removed. Millions of would-be winners were ready to let obsession go, and God or their Higher Power didn't disappoint them.

## Discouragement

PWCPs get discouraged. They've been disappointed so many times, they're bitter. Many have been promised much and were given very little. After awhile, they just quit trying. The person suffering from chronic pain can't afford to quit, yet that is an attitude he or she must be willing to relinquish.

## Fear of Letting Go

It's frightening for some of us to think about giving

up our character defects. It can represent downright terror. Some "addictionologists" are convinced that heroin addiction is as much an addiction to the lifestyle as to heroin. Drinkers love the camaraderie and conviviality around the bar. Giving it up means big changes in lifestyle. Cocaine addicts also must make big changes. Many of their so-called friends have to go. PWCPs also must be willing to give up conduct they're not proud of. Not taking responsibility has to go. Not exercising must go. The shifting of blame must go. The total dependency on others must go. The isolation must go. The bitterness must go. The dropping out of life must go. These are but a few of the things you must be willing to let go of if such things exist in your life right now. Let go, and let God.

## Shopping List

It probably will do no good to present God or your Higher Power with a shopping list. Picking and choosing is not what Step 6 encompasses. You won't get far keeping this character defect and letting go of that one. Bargaining with your Higher Power does not seem like a very good idea. If you have intractable pain you need to be willing to go to any lengths to change anything that may help.

## No Incentive

Many people do not seem to make it because they are not hurting enough. If the hurt is not bad enough, there is no incentive to change. We see adolescents with significant drug problems, but they really have not suffered much...yet. Many mothers and fathers pick up the pieces unendingly, generally out of love, not allowing their children to experience the consequences of their own actions. There is little or no motivation for the adolescent to stop if there are no consequences for his or her actions.

## Desperation

When you are hurt enough, you become desperate for solutions. Desperate people do not ruminate over their defects of character. Desperate people are willing to do anything that is reasonable, as long as it helps.

The word *defect* comes from the Latin *deficere*, meaning to undo or fail. It means lack of something necessary for completeness. It implies shortcomings, weaknesses, flaws, or blemishes. Once identified, these defects must go; they get in the way of good mental health. A PWCP must become tough. Things that weaken resolve must become things of the past. Blemishes must be polished. The Sixth Step is a definitive exercise stating without equivocation that you are ready to let God get rid of all those distracting defects standing in the way of your getting well.

## ▲ STEP 7

Humbly asked Him to remove our shortcomings.

To be humble means to have or show a consciousness of your defects or shortcomings. Step 5 was an admission of your shortcomings and Step 6 confirmed your readiness to turn them over. Now, Step 7 is an instruction to ask Him to remove them... humbly.

### Humility

Humility, humility, humility. If the Steps aren't busy addressing honesty, they're tackling humility. The message seems clear enough. Without humility, you get nowhere. Step 7 begins with the word "humbly." Perhaps the secret of the whole Twelve Step program's success is humility.

## Good Pride

However, pride (the reverse of humility), like pain, is not all bad. We all should take pride in our work, family, home, country, appearance, accomplishments, etc. It's okay to be proud, within reason. A PWCP can certainly be proud of doing the previous six Steps! Pride may be taken in the positive changes made so far. That's good hard-earned, reasonable pride. Pride only becomes ominous when it gets carried away, when it begins to foul up your life. Mark Twain remarked once that "the height of conceit is that point which occurs right before the fall."

## Bad Pride

The undesirable side of pride is well recognized when prestige, material goods, saving face, looking good, and other superficial traits take precedence over spiritual values. Egocentricity begins to rear its decidedly homely head. Successful professionals, men and women in business, people who give orders (not take them), the Type A personalities (who always seem to end up on top) and hard-driving, unrelenting people quite often have little or no humility. Some of those same people develop chronic pain, too. Without humility, it feels degrading to ask for help to remove shortcomings. Without humility, there are probably few, if any, admitted shortcomings. People who lack humility are generally not concerned about God's will; they are concerned about their own wills. They are not about to take advice; they prefer to give it. They aren't working a program; they're running a program. They're not listening; they're talking. They'll die with their chronic pain because they want everything on their terms. It's highly unlikely they will have much time for a Higher Power. People with their own agendas do not go far in the program.

Proud people need no help. They don't need support. They can do it themselves. They don't need God. They don't need anyone. Proud people have their own unique view of reality. Groups are for the weak. Their pain is different, and far worse than the pain of anyone else who has suffered. No one can possibly fathom how badly they hurt. Doctors are dunces, insurance companies are thieves, lawyers are leeches, and the clergy are a bunch of phonies!

Yes, it's safe to say that pride can destroy a program. Can a proud person admit that chronic pain may have left him or her one card short of a full deck when it comes to sanity? If your elevator doesn't go all the way to the top and everyone around you has noticed it for some time, something is very wrong. If you're proud, you're the last one to recognize you're not operating on all eight cylinders. A humble person is willing to ask for and accept help. A humble person is able to ask God from the bottom of the heart to remove shortcomings.

## Spirituality

Not all people who suffer intense, continuous pain are irascible, but many are. Acute pain is enough to drive you around the bend, and chronic pain is even worse. Where do you find the strength and courage, if blinded with pain, to humbly ask God to take away your shortcomings? This is precisely where "spirituality" takes over, and perhaps humility plays a substantial part in it. We keep hearing about the "grace of God"; perhaps that's what happens. Acute pain skillfully applied will make the strongest soldier confess to almost any crime. Chronic pain can level the strongest person, too. Chronic pain is roughly acute pain that never goes away. It's obviously going to take a very powerful force to intervene and make significant changes. Perhaps if you have the humility to ask God to release the floodgates, and really believe it will happen, it will happen. Perhaps if you believe strongly enough, you'll win the spiritual lottery. It may not be accompanied by a roll of thunder and a bolt of lightning, but many people in a Twelve Step program certainly do buy lock, stock, and barrel the value of the spiritual aspect of the program.

Spirituality pertains to much more than having an open telephone line to God. Spirituality spills over into your life. Spirituality seems to drive the whole program. It flows from one CPA member to the next. Goodness seems to replace rancor and hate; sullenness, by infectious laughter and good times; impatience, by patience and stoicism; meanness, by love; and pride, by humility.

## Grace of God

People in the program aren't perfect. Some try, but never seem to change much. Some make great strides and then slip. Some are sober and abstinent with little quality of sobriety. All Anonymous groups are composed of people just like us, normal human beings, striving to make great changes. Imperfections are not shed overnight. With God's grace, most people make great strides. Spirituality is·very real to them. The "grace of God" is very real to them. "There I go but for the grace of God" isn't a platitude to them. The grace of God allows them to decide what shortcomings they possess and gives them the humility to ask God to remove them. They really believe, down deep where it counts, that He will. Even the most embittered PWCP couldn't help but be touched by doing his or her best in performing the Seventh Step. The Sixth Step provided a period of reflection. After due consideration, the person in chronic pain said they were ready to step forward and be counted. In

Step 7, the PWCP asks the Supreme Being, the Higher Power, God, to remove his or her faults, shortcomings, imperfections, defectiveness, deficiencies, inadequacies, fallibility, foibles, etc. What a profoundly spiritual experience! A PWCP needs this kind of spiritual boost. Any small boost helps, but God is not known for being miserly.

## Relief

Removing your shortcomings is like dropping a bag of rocks. People readily admit they sense a feeling of elation, of lightness. Many describe a successful Seventh Step as the lifting of a remarkably heavy burden from their shoulders. A spiritual awakening, or whatever it is, makes them feel good. This type of happiness can't be purchased with money. It has nothing to do with material goods. Many spend hours trying to put feelings into words without much success. Most wish there were some way to keep the powerful sense of relief forever. This is possibly one of those few moments in life when you are closer than ever before to being in the Divine's presence. Having your shortcomings removed is truly a marvelous gift.

## Sublime Experience

It's well accepted by people who specialize in chronic pain that a peaceful, orderly, and comfortable mind greatly influences pain. Doing a good Seventh Step is usually a sublime experience with few rivals. Your focus is changed. When chronic pain is present, any distraction helps. Laughter helps, but it's transient; the removal of your shortcomings, however, is solid stuff. It's difficult to imagine how you couldn't be better, more relaxed, more confident, and more in love with your Higher Power and others after this experience.

## ▲ STEP 8

Made a list of all persons we had harmed, and became *willing* to make amends to them all.

### List

"Making a list of all persons we had harmed" is a project in itself; "being willing to make amends" to all of them takes intestinal fortitude of heroic proportions. If that's not difficult enough, it implies that present relations with those we love should also be improved. It doesn't specifically state that, but when setting out to make amends for transgressions in the past, there's an automatic tendency to clean up the present. The Eighth Step is an ongoing process, and an extremely positive one. It's a real commitment.

### Hurting Others

It's very easy to harm those around you when you're feeling pain. There's a natural tendency to lash out and hurt those closest to you. The old song "You Always Hurt the One You Love" takes on new meaning. It's very hard for people in constant pain not to leave human wreckage in their wake. Trying to make amends to those left in that wake is a lot to ask, but it needs to be done. At least we must be willing to try.

Interpersonal warfare and turmoil are hard on the nervous system. Destructive mental combat does horrible things to this extremely sophisticated, sensitive, and specialized tissue. The nervous system, particularly the central nervous system, carries pain impulses by the billions back and forth all day and night like a giant computer. With pain there's already too much traffic. Interpersonal warfare creates turmoil and it takes the nervous system and throws it against the wall. The closer the relationship, the more the hurt will impact on the central nervous system.

When you harm another, there's a price to be paid, and the price is steep for the PWCP. Disturbed and destructive relationships fuel the already-raging pain communication system. People suffering from chronic pain need equanimity, not turmoil.

## Why Make Amends?

Why not leave the bodies where they're buried? Only a masochist would be interested in trying to mend broken fences! Why resurrect bad memories and hurts? Wouldn't it just rattle the nervous system even more? Wouldn't it make things even worse? It's relatively easy to see how defense mechanisms kick in: denial, intellectualization, suppression, projection, rationalization, and delusions come to the forefront. They allow you to do nothing and stay sick. No one wishes to think about people they have harmed, much less go back and make an attempt to patch things up. Sometimes a PWCP can make Scrooge look good. People in pain have much to rage over. "It isn't fair!" They didn't ask for the pain. Suppressed rage makes a human being miserable. Not dealing with the specific issue of harm done to others, however, keeps you sick.

We are social beings. We don't live in a vacuum. Each day we come in contact with hundreds of people we learn to love or hate, and sometimes a little of each. When you hurt, it's extremely easy for your personal relationships to be in shambles. Most people can take just so much and then they come unglued. When the fire is returned, so often the PWCP can't handle it. It's a vicious cycle of anger, hurt and retaliation, and the pain gets worse. It will drive your friends and family away.

## Not Easy

If you're conscientious, your list of harmed people may be formidable. Many of them may not be God's gift to humanity, either. They may not be very lovable. It takes a good man or woman, plus a generous boost from a Higher Power, to be willing to approach someone who is not friendly or likable and make amends. No one ever said this Step would be easy. You can always fall back and "call headquarters"—prayer can make a big difference. God always seems to be there when you need help. Spirituality seems to come flowing in when people get stuck, but you first have to put in the request for help.

## Earning Tranquility

Most people in AA have an inner peace if they truly work their program. They don't flaunt it. It's there, but not by accident. They earned it. They made a list of those they somehow harmed and they were willing to approach every last one of them and make amends. Inner peace and tranquility did not come easily. Many people frankly admit that the most important factor in bringing them to the various Anonymous organizations is the sight of a group of smiling people having a good time with a sense of peace. Not all Twelve Step members have it, but most are striving for it.

## Clear Conscience

There's something very special and fine about having a clear conscience. People with a clear conscience feel good. They tend to like themselves, and it shows. They like the people around them. Step Eight helps create a clear conscience. Most people are sensitive about wrongs perpetrated on others. They're sensitive because it bothers and worries them. They may suppress the knowledge of the damage inflicted on another, but that leads to poor mental health. The attic needs to be cleaned out; the secrets, the shame, and the hurt need to be fixed. When another human being has been wronged, an attempt to right the wrong must be made.

## Guilt

Guilt is a painful feeling of self-reproach resulting from a belief that we have done something wrong or immoral. It eats away at your soul. It makes you miserable and unhappy. It drives you to do irrational things and keeps you sick. You need to unload it. If one person wrongs another, he or she carries that mental baggage around forever and it gets heavy. When you dump that guilt by at least being willing to make amends, it goes a long way toward establishing better mental health. A PWCP has enough mental and physical burdens. The load needs to be lightened. Being willing to make amends may not completely alleviate the guilt, but it can go a long way. It can't help but brighten the disposition. Just the willingness, the ability to keep putting forth the effort, will make you feel better.

## The Family

People closest to you are likely to have suffered most. The family unit is a good place to start cleaning house. Chronic pain promotes sick family relationships—not always, but often. Arguments, finger pointing, violence, bitterness, accusations, hate, discourtesy, offensiveness, and cursing are all part of the scene. When you are in pain, you have a tendency to lash out and hurt others; sometimes you go for the jugular. Family members know each other well. They can easily tear each other apart. Criticisms may cut deeply. When they fire, they know where to aim and where it hurts the most.

For all these reasons, a good place to start a list of harmed persons is on the home front. Being willing to make amends is an example of love. It seldom goes unnoticed and unappreciated. Spirituality may again save the day. Harmony returns when love flows freely among family members. The PWCP thrives in that kind of family atmosphere. Changing from a life regularly torn by family conflict to a family atmosphere of understanding and helpfulness will produce minor miracles. This may not happen overnight, but being wiling to make amends is a step in the right direction.

## Harm

To "harm" means to cause pain or torment, hurt or injury. It may be physical or mental or both. Gossip can be destructive. Sharp intellects can be used with surgical precision when it comes to doing the other guy in. It's not unusual to see someone in pain inflict suffering on others around them. It's an "If I'm hurting, everyone around me is going to hurt too" syndrome. It's likely the PWCP doesn't realize it, but it can wreak havoc in the lives of those trying to help. If others get hurt too often, they don't come back. After getting your list made, you'll find a great deal of work ahead of you. You will find you may have harmed many people, mostly inadvertently, as a backlash from the hellish torment of pain.

## Ongoing Process

The Eighth Step is ongoing. It's not a one-shot deal. It's a process lasting as long as you work your program. If the PWCP straightens up, then comes up with the list, and in turn, is perfectly willing to make amends, it represents the first of many such exercises in the future. A good member of any Anonymous organization goes through this same process many times over a lifetime.

## Will to Make it Right

"Will" is the power of making a reasoned choice or decision, or of controlling your own actions. Step 8 suggests making a reasoned choice to make amends. The willingness to use that power springs from within. When your head is on straight and well-lubricated by God's grace, you become willing to right many things, to look at the past and search carefully for how your actions may have harmed others, and to examine the present. Once the list is determined, the PWCP can look with both trepidation and courage to a future time when amends can be made.

## Honesty

Perhaps the most important things to remember in Step 8 is the all-powerful and pervasive word *honesty*. A dishonest person will come with 10,000 defense mechanisms for whittling away at the list of those who have been wronged. A dishonest person will develop criteria so broad that anything short of murder will not qualify as harm. They weasel out of the Eighth Step by intellectualizing and rationalizing every bad thing they ever did. They spend most of their time adjusting their halos. Their list will be blatantly devoid of names. An honest list will include the names of those who've been damaged, for whatever reason, by the one who knows deeply that a significant wrong was perpetrated. Your conscience comes into play, and the worse the transgression, the more uneasy you become. Honesty, honesty, honesty—the Eighth Step is dictated by honesty! The more you sweat over this one, the better the Step. A cursory effort equals a poor to mediocre result.

## Sponsor

Consulting a sponsor always helps. A good sponsor will usually be able to see through the defense mechanisms and get you back on track. Chronic Pain Anonymous, as with all Anonymous organizations, contains a host of wise people who understand. They understand how easy it is to kid yourself into doing a weak Eighth.

Groups frequently split into Step meetings where each Step is carefully dissected, analyzed, argued, and digested. Often a sponsor will direct his or her charge to a specific Step meeting. If you're fortunate and privileged enough to attend a discussion of the Eighth Step, it may solve some perplexing questions, particularly in the definition of "harm." Anonymous members seem to flow back and forth between all organizations, so attending a good AA Step meeting will probably suffice if none is available in CPA. As a bigger organization, AA offers a greater number of Step meetings.

## ▲ STEP 9

Made direct amends to such people wherever possible, except when to do so would injure them or others.

### Direct Amends

Direct amends means just that. Essentially, in The Twelve Steps, "direct" means a one-to-one meeting. It's a task few people relish. Because it can be distasteful, some people choose to skip it. The other Steps can be handled, but when it comes to a face-to-face encounter or a direct phone call, they chicken out. They find it "too hard" to do, too much to ask. They may pick one or two easy marks on their list, but the sticky cases are deferred to another time and place.

## Difficulty

The Ninth Step doesn't allow you to be highly selective. If someone has been wronged, amends should be made. It matters little if you can't stand the offended party. Chances are, many of the people on your list are not your favorite people, but the issue isn't likes and dislikes. If you have committed a wrong, you should make a serious attempt to right that wrong. "Going to any lengths" has an ominous ring. You must muster grit at times, and this is one of those times. The Ninth Step scares off some pretty tough customers. A macho guy has a difficult time saying "I'm sorry." A proud person chokes on each word. A dishonest person never gets around to it at all. The weak run away from the task. It takes a great amount of humility plus an abundance of courage to say "I'm sorry." Granted, it's easier if you like the person in question, but it's still not a comfortable matter.

## Do It!

Step 9 requires no debate. The deliberation and scrutinizing were done in Eight. Nine is the consequent action. They have a saying in AA about "walking your talk." You learn to walk your talk. Talk is cheap, and doing what you'll say you'll do is often quite different. Step 9 is for strong people, and PWCPs have to be strong. Years of pain weaken you physically and mentally, but you must find the strength somewhere. CPA is a font of strength for you, and the ultimate resource, of course, is always your Higher Power. If you don't get bogged down by pride, you usually find the strength to get the job done. The spiritual nature of the program seems to make it happen.

## Timing and Prudence

You don't have to face the entire list of people you've harmed all at once. Each name may take several different peacemaking meetings or phone calls. Nothing in the Steps seems to be etched in stone. Timing might be an issue. Timing requires thoroughness. "Except when to do so would injure them or others" may require some timing. You would be remiss to approach an injured one when they're vulnerable. Prudence is a virtue. Prudence is the ability to exercise sound judgment in practical matters. Don't try to make amends in a crowd of noisy people, for instance—that wouldn't be sound judgment. Avoid embarrassing the offended person— don't use the newspaper, radio, or television to make amends! Common sense rules the day.

### Fear

Fear gets in the way of a good Ninth Step. You'll somehow have to overcome your fear of embarrassing yourself or feeling degraded, humiliated, awkward, mortified, or disconcerted over having to approach the offended people on your list. PWCPs know all about fear. They fear they'll never get well. They fear the next surgery. They fear they'll not be able to live without narcotics. Some are even afraid they'll live, not die. They know what fear is all about! Still, when it comes to overriding their pride, some dig in their heels. They choke on their pride, and can't find the courage to make amends to certain people.

The fear of rejection is a problem. It's not pleasant, but people live through it. If you're trying to make amends and are told where to go, it doesn't do much for your ego. It's an unusual happening, but the world is full of imperfect people. People who experience chronic pain have experienced their share of rejection. Most have been rejected by physicians, physical therapists, insurance companies, state compensation—you name it. (When physicians give it their best shot and fail, it bothers them, too. Physicians aren't known for having small egos. When nothing works, most refer PWCPs to psychiatrists with the inference that "It's all in your head!") With a long record of rejection, it's small wonder the PWCP is gun-shy, but don't let the fear of rejection keep you from even trying to make amends.

## Feeling Good

Like most processes, once you make your list and have some experience making amends, it gets easier. Most amends turn out very well, with both parties expressing warm feelings. Miraculous healing doesn't take place, but it certainly makes you sense something good has happened. It does wonders for your disposition, and the good feelings can be infectious. People who omit the Ninth Step make a big mistake. The ones who "went for it" are happy they did.

## ▲ STEP 10

Continued to take a personal inventory, and when we were wrong, promptly admitted it.

The Twelve Steps are a way of life. This is particularly true of the Tenth Step. You might speculate that all previous Steps are simply a preparation for the Tenth. Each Step is predicated on the last. People have tried to rearrange them, change the wordings and make revisions, but in the end they remain the same as they were when they were written in the 1930s.

## Continued Inventory

The Tenth Step is a declaration that all the preceding work doesn't end. The personal inventory is to be continued and, if you feel you've committed a transgression, you have to admit it. A strict and exhaustive inventory took place in Step 4, the exact nature of wrongs was admitted to God and another person in Step 5, and a decision to move toward health was reached in Step 6. You actually ask God or your Higher Power for the removal of character defects in Step 7, a list of wronged people was prepared in Step 8, and making amends was undertaken in Step 9.

Everything flows right along. The Tenth Step is a resolution to keep the flow moving. It's a resolution to keep a beautiful philosophy of life afloat. Self-inventory and self-evaluation are to be your lifelong pursuits.

## Grateful Victims

Since the inception of AA, people who love the philosophy of Anonymous organizations have been saying they're grateful they fell victim to their addiction. That's a startling bit of information. It's akin to being grateful for developing carcinoma. Because of their addiction, they became exposed to the philosophy of AA or some other Anonymous group. If they had not succumbed to their addiction, they would never have been privy to the tenets of the Twelve Steps. The Tenth Step is an integral part of that philosophy.

Old habits, like old soldiers, never die. They just fade away. They rarely disappear with a wave of a magic wand. When you work Step 10, you work to assure that old habits keep fading away. The people who wrote the Steps knew much about human nature. They left little to chance. The inventory and amends were recognized as real jewels to help keep members on track, and members were encouraged to take an inventory and make amends daily. They were not much for one big fling. They wanted to avoid being static; they strove for constant improvement.

## Patterns

When you do a daily inventory, patterns emerge. You'll uncover bad habits like "acting out," impulsive conduct, lying, refusing to accept responsibility, inveterate whining and complaining, blaming others, refusing to exercise, demanding attention, taxing the family's financial resources, unwarranted criticism of those who make great sacrifices for them, egocentricity, being waited on, not returning favors, showing little or no interest in other family members, being ungrateful, isolating, exhibiting no drive or laughter or love, refusing to perform some type of reasonable work, being a slave to the TV, hanging on to the pills, pushing for more surgery and more hurt, looking everywhere for help except from within—these are but a few of the patterns that sometimes emerge. The Tenth Step directs you to admit these habits and urges you to do something about them.

Here's a story that sheds some further light on this process: "Two men were walking side by side down a road, and one kept stumbling and falling down. Finally, the guy who was getting all beat up asked the other why he never stumbled and fell. The man responded by saying, 'It helps dearly if you look down and avoid the holes and rocks!'" The daily inventory uncovers and discloses the holes and rocks in your path. Learn to walk around the holes and rocks, or you may alternatively choose to keep stumbling and falling. The Tenth, if done properly, points out your problem areas. Falling into holes is nonproductive. God didn't intend it for you.

## Keep It Simple

Some very sick people need professional help when they *look* for the holes and rocks in their lives. They need psychiatric, psychological, or pastoral help. There's an old saying: "If it's incomprehensible, it's mathematical; if it doesn't make any sense at all, it's either economics or psychology." The point is that the human mind is extremely complex. Sometimes professionals seem to muddy the waters and turn little problems into big problems. It seems to work better to take big problems and turn them into little problems. Sometimes there are no absolute answers. It's often better not to worry about everything, just work the Twelve Steps and see what happens. Keep it simple. Give it a year or so. But seek professional help if the simple approach doesn't work.

## Negativity Down, Optimism Up

A PWCP can get down on himself or herself without much effort. Negativity may become a way of life, but negativity has to go. The Tenth Step is a wonderful mechanism to use in order to accomplish that particular task. With the Tenth, you'll begin to see change, positive change. You'll find out you can accept responsibility for making yourself well. You'll find yourself being grateful to people who go the extra mile for you. You'll see how you still have the mental and physical assets for helping yourself. You'll discover you can still laugh at yourself (and others). PWCPs can quit being isolated and perhaps get a new CPA group going if their group becomes too large. They notice as time goes on that life is indeed worth living again.

Negative feelings cause stress, and PWCPs need to learn how to deal with stress. Again, the properly-done inventory points out the holes and rocks so you can learn to walk abound them. The daily inventory brings to your attention the people and circumstances that create stress. If a recognizable pattern develops, you can avoid it.

## Eliminating Stress

Stress comes from the Latin *strictus*. In English it means a mental or physical tension or strain. Tension and strain mentally and physically overload the system. The load needs reduction, so try anything that releases tension. Biofeedback, relaxation techniques, osteopathic manipulation, chiropractic treatment and/or acupuncture—if it helps relieve stress, use it. "God helps those who help themselves." When you feel stress is developing, the inventory may point out a pattern of circumstances contributing to it. It's time to develop a strategy to prevent it.

Everyone has stress in their lives. Even before a PWCP became a PWCP, life was full of stress! Some people forget that. The PWCP's problem now is a live-wire, super-sensitive nervous system that doesn't sleep. Normal daily stresses can grow out of proportion. Schemes and stratagems can be devised to either avoid the stress altogether or reduce it when it occurs. A daily inventory puts you in touch with the when, how, where, and how stressful incidents occur. If you're unaware that a problem exists, you can't fight it. Pain is definitely aggravated by stress, and the PWCP isn't looking for more pain—anything that helps lighten the load will be welcomed with open arms.

## When To Do It

You don't have to do the inventory at a specific time, but most choose a time just before turning in at night. Some people fall asleep every night performing the Tenth. Sleep is very hard to achieve for someone in chronic pain, so going over the day's inventory beats counting sheep, and it's much more productive. It provides ample time to examine the day's happenings and ruminate over destructive patterns. There are many rocks to stumble over or holes to fall into in a PWCP's day. The daily inventory is truly a spiritual exercise, too. You would think God or a Higher Power would look favorably upon the person who goes over the day's inventory every night before going to sleep. You would think God would be much more likely to share His beneficence with people who work hard on their programs.

## Learn To Handle Bad Feelings

One of the real pluses in doing the daily inventory before sleep is it seems to foster the release of feelings. PWCPs perceive pain all day and night, and emotional feelings are hard to describe and weed out from the pain. Going over the inventory, feelings play a large part in the affects of the happenings of the day. Disappointments make us feel bad. Warfare with a spouse or partner makes us feel low. Good news and good experiences help balance things. If good things happen, the pain is usually not as bad. Bad experiences rattle the nervous system and create internal chaos. You can't avoid bad experiences; they come with living. You can, however, learn from them. An inventory helps you discern a reasonable way of handling those bad feelings with the least amount of friction. Any reduction in the stress level helps. The inventory helps you prepare a good plan of action, and that plan of action helps you to be prepared, alert, and clear-witted for the next experience. It helps keep a lid on your central nervous system.

Counselors like to spend a good part of their lives encouraging people to show their feelings. Behavior is equated with how you really are inside. Blunted, flat "affect" is interpreted as very little going on inside. If someone relates a terrible experience with no "affect," it's interpreted as not meaning very much to them. Unless feelings are displayed that coincide on the same level with the incident, the event is perceived as less important, or the person relating it is temporarily or permanently deranged.

Depression, schizophrenia, or mania alter the display of feelings. Counselors often have difficulty sorting it all out. They rely heavily on exhibited feelings. Feelings are an important part of life. Friends, family, and fellow CPA members react to your show of emotions. Temper tantrums drive people away; expressing feelings of solicitation and love bring people closer together. The daily inventory helps remind you of how important it is to let others know what is going on inside. Not allowing others to get to know you is not good. The daily inventory helps guard you against not showing appropriate emotions not allowing others to fairly judge how good or how miserable you feel.

## Mental and Physical Health

Good mental health promotes good physical health. It's important for the PWCP to understand this. Anyone who suffers from chronic pain should be struggling constantly for improved mental and physical health. Since the mind strongly influences the body, it makes sense to strive for equanimity. The inventory helps do that.

## Resentments

The Tenth Step helps get rid of resentment, and resentment has to go. Resentment is a feeling (there's that word again!) of displeasure and indignation from a sense of being injured or offended. People with chronic pain tend to have "thin skins." When someone hurts all the time, it doesn't take very much to incur their displeasure and indignation. They raise exquisite antennas. People resent all kinds of things: being impoverished, unloved, not being promoted, or doing more than their share of work. They resent being dumped on for no reason, not being more gifted intellectually, or being in constant pain. Resentment is like a spreading cancer, coloring and souring the disposition. It severely restricts your ability to think and plan ahead. It primes your temper. Not much good comes from resentment—it's a slow poison. Step 10 is a daily mental housecleaning chore. If resentment is dealt with every day, there's no build-up, and that's good for the PWCP. When you accumulate resentment, your pain tends to get worse in response. The daily inventory forces you to deal with it, defuse it, and hopefully get rid of it. When resentments are discarded every night, you'll sleep better and awaken more refreshed.

## Priorities

A nightly inventory promotes a shift of priorities for you. Personal wealth, prestige, and power are familiar goals in our society. Unfortunately, there's a proclivity to get carried away with acquiring material goods, and it soon replaces the pursuit of spiritual values. The PWCP doesn't want to end up as the richest man or woman in the cemetery. The Steps don't advocate poverty or running away from power, but they don't embrace blind ambition either. The nightly inventory helps you keep things in perspective. If you keep current with the inventory process, it will help you keep your values straight.

## Accurate Inventory

"When we were wrong" encompasses interesting territory. It implies good judgment, for one thing. It assumes you have a sound mind to judge objective facts and therefore draw fair conclusions. Be careful not to be too righteous in the inventory. It's been said the world is divided into two kinds of people, the righteous and the unrighteous, and the righteous are the ones who do the dividing. So when doing the daily inventory, you may need some help. A sponsor or fellow CPA member might help sift through the facts and keep the inventory as accurate as possible.

The Tenth Step provides a mechanism to keep life on the straight and narrow. It's a beautiful, magnificent piece of advice. It allows you to mull over your conflicts, delve into the whys and wherefores of your daily life, weigh your conflicts, prepare for future crises, etc. With God's grace, it will make your life more pleasant and serene. A PWCP can certainly use that.

## ▲ STEP 11

Sought through prayer and meditation to improve our conscious contact with God, as we *understood* Him, praying only for knowledge of His will for us and the power to carry that out.

### Prayer and Meditation

The PWCP, the alcoholic, or any addict for that matter, doesn't seem to get very far trying to slug it out alone. They need help. Step 11 recommends asking for that help from God "as we understood Him." It recommends prayer and meditation.

### Blaming God

God frequently gets blamed for everything by people in chronic pain. No one will ever know why they have been singled out to suffer. Looking around, a PWCP can be filled with much anger and resentment when comparing himself or herself with others. Often people with chronic pain have little money, no self-respect, and a bleak future. They can make themselves extremely miserable wallowing in negativity. God is a fairly big target, so there's a decided tendency to unload on Him.

There are so many things we don't understand. We can't understand why God permits war with all its horror and debauchery, why He seems to shower worthless people with munificence, why He allows children to be born without limbs, why He "kicks our legs out from under us" periodically, even though we're trying our best. Why? It would be nice to have all the answers, but unfortunately, we don't; we just struggle along, hopefully doing our best. We utilize our assets to the best of our ability, and we try to be grateful for what we have. Fixation on the negative side of the ledger seems to accomplish little except to make things worse. The person suffering with chronic pain needs to look at the brightest side of the ledger, where light falls. When going around all day afraid to move the wrong way, afraid to cough, afraid to walk any distance, afraid of temperature changes, or afraid to do anything to aggravate the pain, it's difficult to look at the bright side. Help is needed.

### Prayer

Prayer is simply communication with God—He talks with us. Step 11 suggests you get busy and start the dialogue. He obviously has some big plans for you. He directs your every action. He knows your past and future. Unfortunately, about the only time most people get very excited about God is when the train comes off the track. Step 11 does not say anything about praying only when you're in trouble. Step 11 specifically states you should maintain regular communication. It implies that you become theocentric instead of egocentric.

### Knowledge and His Will

Apparently God is not into filling orders. If God gave you everything you asked for, you would spend your waking hours on your knees. Everyone has had the experience of having prayed hard for something, had their prayers answered and then, sometime in the future, wished He had not granted the request. The founding fathers of AA suggested in the Eleventh Step that people pray only for "knowledge of His will for us." That message clearly connotes not your will, but God's. Again, egocentricity is cast aside. When things get dumped into our laps that don't coincide with our wants, however, we begin to question God's wisdom. The Eleventh Step emphatically states that we pray for knowledge and the ability to understand His will for us, but it takes humility to accept God's will. Essentially, you're asked to play the cards God has dealt you. PWCPs have a difficult time with this concept, and rightly so. They need help.

### Discourse With God

Prayer and meditation is hard to come by when you're in pain. Pain is distracting. Advice such as "offer it up" doesn't go over well when you're sweating blood. Pain relief is wanted, not advice. Unfortunately, total relief and obliteration of pain is next to impossible for PWCPs. Intractable pain means just that—it's not going to go away. You must learn to live with it, finding ways to make inroads through the pain, grabbing at any slight measure that lightens your burden. Difficult as it is, you must try to take the focus away from the pain. A time-honored way of doing that is to open a discourse with God or your Higher Power. Therein lies not total relief, but a definite step in the right direction.

### Keep It Simple

Many people with large intellects, actual or imagined, seem to run into a brick wall when it comes to prayer and meditation. If they're presented with something they can't touch, measure, count, weigh, or see under a microscope, they're not interested. They can't see God, and unless He sends telegrams or visits them personally or leaves them with stigmata, they can't bring themselves to even try praying. "Praying is for fools." They don't have the time for it. They develop all sorts of defenses which allow them not to exercise the prayer and meditation option. This only complicates things beyond belief. An old priest who had about five degrees once described prayer as simply settling back in the old La-Z-Boy and having a "heart to heart" with God. He was also an avid AA member, fond of saying "Keep it simple!" Intellectuals do anything but keep it simple. Many seem to prefer to keep it complicated. Talking with God is simple. It helps, and it's a major source of power and strength. People who suffer constant pain need all the power and strength they can get their hands on. They need to communicate with God.

## Meditation

Meditation is a marvelous source of peace and tranquility. To "meditate" means to reflect upon or study. You need not take an option on a cave in a nearby mountain to meditate. All that's needed is a quiet place with few distractions. A church is great, the woods are wonderful, but any room that's restful and softly lit will be fine. Withdraw from the world, with all its cares, and ponder what's going on in your life. This time-out period can be done any time during the day, but it's essential to make a specific time for it. For a PWCP, it's invaluable time.

Tons of literature have been produced on the subject of meditation. If the subject was of little import, it's likely there would be little interest. Men and women who devote their lives exclusively to God spend much time in meditation. The Eleventh does not request seeking solace in a monastery or convent. Those who developed the Twelve Steps just recognized the power of meditation and recommended it.

One interesting, peaceful counselor used to spend an hour a day in meditation. He would arrive for work in his Arizona hospital at five o'clock every morning and spend one hour meditating in his office. He was a recovering alcoholic with a doctorate in psychology. He was a brilliant counselor, with great equanimity. He figured morning meditation provided the spiritual fuel to get him through the day. He is with his Maker now, but a more competent, caring, and spiritual man never walked this earth. Meditation was a simple time commitment for him, a small amount of time that yielded daily rewards.

Time limits aren't crucial with meditation. Spend a few minutes, ten or fifteen minutes—there's good reason to suspect God is more interested in quality than quantity. A brief ten minutes pilfered from daily TV time should do the trick. Meditation definitely makes you slow down, smell the flowers, count blessings, rise above daily strife, evaluate priorities, listen, learn, relax, chat, and visit with your Higher Power. PWCPs need to learn to commune with their spiritual source. They have a dire need for quiet introspection. Once the habit is established, most say the experience helps them dearly. They say it recharges their spiritual batteries. If anything helps alleviate the pain, you should happily try it! Meditation certainly seems to be a great source of strength.

## Power

Perhaps the key to the Eleventh Step is the word "power," as in "the power to carry that out." PWCPs are asked to pray for the knowledge of His will, but also for the power to carry it out. Power means the ability to produce or to affect strongly. Pray for illumination about what God has in mind for you, but also for the ability to get the job done. Chronic pain can drain a person completely. It seems when pain is part of the equation, less and less is able to be accomplished. "Carrying out God's will" gets dumped, thrown in with the general ennui often typifying the amount of energy expended by people whose lives are governed by pain. Mental and physical action is minimal. Exercise is ruled out. Life is relegated to monitoring TV. There isn't much power, there isn't much activity, but there's a crying need for change. It takes power to perform God's will. It takes power to change negative attitudes. You may be able to fathom God's will, but embracing it is another matter. The Eleventh Step suggests that you pray for that power.

Someone once noted sarcastically that in order to get a loan from a bank, you must first prove you don't need it. It's reasonable to assume God is a very good banker, and He will dispense His power when and where it will do the most good. Material goods may not be what's best; alleviation of some of the pain might be better. A Rolls Royce would probably not be a justifiable request. Asking for the courage to follow through with things learned from a physical therapist in a chronic pain management unit would probably be appropriate. Asking God to make you a better husband and father would be reasonable. Regardless of specifics, one thing is for sure—just ask!

## Proximity to God

Once the process of praying becomes a reality, most people experience a closeness with God. Other people will take note because the PWCP will begin to act differently. Power flows from the powerful, and the most powerful is your Higher Power. A sense of security is a blessing experienced by those who walk with God. Walking in concert with God brings back a spring in the step and a warm glow to the heart. Union with God is the ultimate job. Theologians describe heaven as final union with God.

People who are close to God seem to radiate an inner beauty. They have an inner peace. Prayer and meditation will bring you closer to God. Time invested in prayer and meditation may be the most valuable and profitable of your entire day. The Eleventh Step promotes a proximity to God by encouraging the process to start. And keep it simple! Prayer is just spiritual conversation.

## ▲ STEP 12

Having had a spiritual awakening as the result of these Steps, we tried to carry this message to others and to practice these principles in all our affairs.

### Review

Let's briefly review. In Step 1, there's an admission of powerlessness and unmanageability. Step 2 states there's a Higher Power that can restore us to sanity. Step 3 is a "turning over" of both will and life to God. Step 4 is an inventory. Step 5 is about admission to God and to another human being. Step 6 is preparation for the Seventh, a request for God to remove all shortcomings. Step 8 makes us develop a list of people we have offended for the purpose of making amends. Step 9 is about making the amends. Step 10 encourages a continuous inventory. Step 11 is a strong recommendation for prayer and meditation.

Step 12 says practice the Principles and pass them along to others.

## Sharing

When something very good comes into your life, the natural tendency is to want to share it. This is particularly true of people with chronic pain, because nothing previously came close to providing relief. If something turns life from abject misery and despair to a sense of well-being and hope, it's most likely a person would want to share the secret. By nature, most of us are truly incompetent secret keepers. Step 12 allows the good news to be shared with others who have the same problem.

## Changes

If PWCPs truly practice the Twelve Steps, it would be difficult for those around them not to notice dramatic changes. You need not be a Sherlock Holmes to recognize the transition from hostility to peacefulness, despair to joy, unpredictability to dependability, and spectator to participant. Nothing happens overnight, but when continuing to work the Steps, your progress is assured. The changes in your life can't be ignored. Curious observers will be prone to ask, "What's happened to you?"

## Patience

Helping others should not be entertained until your sponsor or other CPA members give you the green light. Most of the wiser heads in AA recommend waiting for a year or two before trying to do extended Twelve Step work. Too many have been lost by jumping into the water trying to save another before learning to swim well themselves. They also suggest no major changes for about a year: changes in job, marriage, geographic moves, business decisions, etc. They suggest you spend the first few years concentrating on yourself. If a person in chronic pain sees another's transformation and seeks similar counsel, they should be referred to a stable person with longevity in the program. Be patient, kind, solicitous, and offer moral support, but it's best to refer someone elsewhere until you're given the Twelve Step green light. There's an extremely strong urge to save the world when you're getting better, but it's advised to wait before buckling on a sword.

## Giving

One of the beautiful facets of all Anonymous groups is the innate philosophy of giving. The last Step dramatizes it. Someone who has been spiritually awakened is asked to carry the message to others (when they're ready), and there's nothing said about any reward for doing so. The one delivering the message mustn't expect to get anything in return. It's impossible to thank a good member of any Anonymous group. The same reply is always offered—"Oh, don't thank me; I do it for myself!" The reward is in the giving. What a beautiful philosophy of life.

## Helping Others

Most AA members look forward with great anticipation to participating in Twelve Step work. Helping another member out of the depths of despair is an incomparable feeling. To get someone to his or her first meeting, sponsor another person, witness the gradual transformation, eventually see that same person reaching out to help another—to have played a part, no matter how small, in another's recovery, has to be one of life's great satisfactions. Promotion of Twelve Step work comes in many forms. Beating a drum on the corner is not one of them, however. Showing up at meetings, sharing feelings, offering support and encouragement, and exploring mutual experiences are all forms of Twelve Step work. Setting a positive example is probably the most powerful form of persuasion. Talk is very cheap. Walking the talk is "practicing the Principles."

## Twelve Steps Work

People in chronic pain like to see results—they want to get well and they want it yesterday. Some are so irascible from pain they tend to drive people away; frequently they relate only to someone who "has been there." Recovering PWCPs are special people with great gifts to offer. Precisely because they have suffered in a like manner, they can relate to other sufferers. Perhaps for the first time, a person in intense pain may have a live audience at CPA that understands, not just one person but several. For many it's like walking from a blizzard into a warm room. For the first time, a PWCP is able to sit down and talk to people who have struggled, and continue to struggle, to turn their lives around. They have a unique, beautiful set of principles to follow, a blueprint for the revision and rebuilding of their lives and an association filled with people who comprehend chronic pain. In sharing what God has given them, they're doing Twelve Step work.

## Family Life

A major benefit of the Steps is the carryover into family life. Philosophy isn't left at the meetings. The love shared in the meetings spills over into each member's family life. The family functions better, there's more order, and very often there's an improved financial picture. Love gradually replaces hatefulness and distrust. Family members are incredulous at first. As time progresses, they accept the welcome changes and respond accordingly.

## Relapse

As long as you "practice the Principles," your private spiritual awakening doesn't end and progress is assured. Slacking off, reverting to past conduct, not getting to meetings regularly, getting lazy about exercise, drug-seeking behavior, losing contact with your sponsor, and ignoring prayer and meditation are all sure signs of imminent relapse. (If you decide to be a bodybuilder, you have to do strengthening exercises every day. As months progress, your muscles ripple; slacking off, your muscles turn to flab, and trying to lift a normal amount of weight may tear your muscle tissue.) "Practicing the Principles" keeps your mind healthy, strong, and sharp. When crises hit, you can handle them. Your mind and body are ready. Vigilance comes with working the Principles. If you are vigilant and prepared, it's unlikely you will walk over the edge of a cliff.

## Striving for Perfection

Following the Twelve Steps is a way of striving for perfection. The world is not filled with perfect people and they don't do perfect things. Anonymous organizations aren't filled with perfect people, either. They're populated with "normal" people who are endeavoring to improve their lives by following the Principles and Philosophy developed in the Steps.

Sometimes others equate actions by one Anonymous member as 100% typical of the organization. Sometimes Twelve Step practitioners are subjected to some bizarre conduct within the organization that makes them draw back. If and when this happens, they need to take it to their meetings and not allow it to destroy their own programs. If a member gets carried away by fear or anger, the group will intervene and bring him or her back to earth in a hurry before there's too much damage. It's one of the great strengths of the group process in the Anonymous organizations.

## Two Steppers

Occasionally we run into "Two Steppers." They do a good First Step, then skip the next ten and move on to the Twelfth Step. They go from a recognition of their own disastrous conduct to a new position of trying to rescue every PWCP within their view. They can do considerable damage to themselves, others, and their organization. It's best for you to gain strength gradually by taking each Step as it comes and nurturing it until you're advised to move on. Rome wasn't built in a day, and you are not ready for rescue work in a few weeks or months.

## Life Becomes Livable

When you suffer from chronic pain, there's a marked tendency to drop out and tune out of the human race. Using the Twelve Steps and following the Principles, you are brought back into the fold. Intractable pain doesn't go away; however, by using the Principles you learn to live and manage the pain, and by leaning on CPA, life becomes livable. There is no support quite like the support provided by fellow PWCPs. There is no greater feeling or greater satisfaction than helping others turn their lives around. God or a Higher Power seems to be there when needed. The spiritual awakening resulting from following the Steps conscientiously can't help but spill over in hundreds of ways, influencing everyone and everything in your life. The tumultuous life of a PWCP can use some order and peace.

## Winners

The Twelve Steps provide both order and peace. The mind governs the body, and a more tranquil mind helps you coexist with pain in greater tolerance and acceptance. Millions of men and women have found comfort in following the Twelve Step Principles. A PWCP is an excellent candidate to join the many winners who have used the Principles to their advantage and finally passed them along to others.

# The Twelve

# Traditions

### ▲ Guidelines

The Twelve Traditions are a set of guidelines set down to give additional strength to the Twelve Step program. They're carefully thought-out suggestions of conduct specifically designed to avoid misinterpretation and speculation. They spell out purpose and guidance for those who strive for personal and spiritual growth. They are tried and true, and many Twelve Step members refer to them as the glue that holds the individual groups together.

### Growth

Most groups seem to grow and flourish depending upon how well they adhere to the Twelve Traditions. Obviously the Traditions are for group protection and development. They've been formulated to protect the unique character of all Anonymous organizations.

### Insurance

In a sense, the Traditions direct the group in order to guide and protect the individual members. Guidelines are needed to insure the common welfare. An organization going in twenty directions simultaneously is soon famous for nothing but confusion.

The process goes nowhere and the group soon disintegrates.

### Serious Advice

The Traditions, however, aren't rules and regulations. They're not commandments, but words and phrases communicating serious advice. The Traditions aren't to be taken lightly. Many suggest one be read at the opening of each meeting, to firmly place them in the minds of all members. This practice should convey to everyone the importance assigned to these guidelines. The Traditions need to be studied, weighed, argued, and thoroughly understood.

## ▲ Tradition 1

Our common welfare should come first; personal progress for the greatest number depends on unity.

Unity is the message of the First Tradition. Unity is a common thread finely woven through all the Traditions. Harmony among the members takes very high priority.

### Common Welfare

Chronic Pain Anonymous is comprised of individuals. Each has his or her own thoughts, ideas, and convictions. PWCPs may have a predilection for egocentricity. The world revolves around them, and everything is focused around their pain. Egocentrics are prone to dominate. It's difficult for egocentrics to operate in a group, but operate in a group they must. Individuality has its place, but it must be subjugated to the common good in this organization. Common welfare must be the number one goal. "Personal progress for the greatest number depends on unity"; unity is destroyed by egocentricity. Before he became active in CPA, a member said he used to leave every business meeting convinced everyone in the room had recorded and preserved for posterity every word he had said. That's the type of grandiosity that must go. In CPA, egocentricity must be replaced by common welfare.

### Sharing

Harmonious relationships at CPA mean working together, sharing ideas, respecting the ideas of others, placing other people's feelings ahead of yours, listening attentively, drawing out introverted members, not forcing your will on others, and keeping an open mind; in short, it's being gentlemen and gentlewomen. Harmonious relationships also depend on your willingness to share feelings. One of the real benefits of CPA is the discovery that the majority of members share many of the same fears, problems, likes, dislikes, aspirations, and even friends.

Active members of CPA—your "pain pals"— soon discover they aren't bad people. Introspection sometimes makes you unfairly self-critical. Sharing in a meeting draws pain sufferers from their self-imposed exile, from behind the walls of denial: the reticent become talkative, the meek more assertive, and the shy more forward. CPA is essentially people helping people. By sharing experiences, knowledge is broadened and confidence is restored. The individual member, however, must have the courage to vocalize ideas and feelings. Difficult as it may be, feelings must be expressed. Voyeurs make little progress. Risks must be taken. Troubles need to be unburdened and aired in the group. Honesty keeps you well; bottled up, hostile and angry feelings keep you ill. Each individual needs to air feelings. It cultivates good mental health. Doing this on a one-to-one basis may suffice, but it's much more reward-ing in a group. It's more rewarding because your peers can offer accurate, generous, and beneficial feedback.

## Silence

Retreating into silence is a cop-out. Often the problem tearing you up is the very same problem bothering the person in the next chair. Sharing your troubles may save another member. Others at the meeting may have suffered through the same dilem-mas. The feedback may be tremendously helpful. Just being willing to discuss the problem tends to lighten the burden. Honest, open-minded discus-sion promotes common welfare. It also promotes unity.

## Blowhards

There are some members who will have an opinion about everything. Because they express themselves well, they have a tendency to take over or dominate meetings. Other members compare themselves men-tally to these know-it-all types and are intimidated by them. They retreat further into silence. There always seems to be at least one blowhard running loose at every social gathering; they contradict some, interrupt others, and argue about everything. "I" is their favorite pronoun. Taking a vote, the other members would probably like to have the prima donna bound and gagged.

## Unity and Common Welfare

The common good calls for patience, kindness and fortitude, up to a point. The common good demands good judgment for action taken. Unity is paramount. There are no standard solutions, how-ever. One reason there are so many meetings is that they take on personalities just as people do. One obnoxious individual may eventually end up as the only one at the meeting. Still, we must exercise charity and love—or at least try to help. The First Tradition proclaims very clearly that unity and common welfare are vital and decisions must be weighed with this in mind. Common sense usually dominates decisions with group involvement. As long as the common good is the number one priority, reasonable judgments are commonly made and unity is preserved.

### Rescue

The Higher Power, more often than not, comes to the rescue in sticky situations. Where the Twelve Steps are practiced, He seems to affect tranquility and peace. When called upon, He seems to be a major force in promoting unity. When unity is threatened, it certainly doesn't hurt to "call headquarters." Higher Power has had a good deal of practice in the rescue business.

### Paradox

Some CPA members take umbrage with the fact that the group, the whole, the unity must take preference over the individual. You hear: "By God, I'm my own man. Nobody tells me how to think. I'm no groupie. Individuals built this country. I've always done my own thing." Notice how often the pronoun "I" pops up? CPA is somewhat of a paradox. All the Anonymous groups are. CPA is a group of strong-minded people who individually accept the responsibility for getting well. No one can do it for them. They accept the responsibility themselves, as individuals, and their strength comes from within. If they win, they take the bows. (They are working their own program, so why not?) If they lose, they take the beating. They accept the responsibility. Nonetheless, in spite of all the individuality, they must function in the group.

## Combined Strength

CPA says "Keep your individualism," but subjugate it to the common welfare. By yourself, you've lost and will continue to lose; in the group, your individualism will be strengthened to the point where you can win. God is in your group. The CPA motto is: "He has so much strength that with His help and our common strength, He'll turn you into a winner!" That's not a promise, that's a fact. Combining strengths makes for powerful forces; suddenly the paradox becomes understandable and viable. The individual soon learns to muzzle personal desires for common good. That's personal growth. Wealth, power, and prestige take a back seat. Every thought and action is mitigated by how it affects the other members. Thoughtlessness is replaced by thoughtfulness. The more members give, the more they get. And you can't help but think that God must play a big hand in all of it.

## ▲ Tradition 2

For our group purpose, there is but one authority—a loving God as He may express Himself in our group conscience. Our leaders are but trusted servants; they do not govern.

## Group Conscience

Group conscience is merely majority decision. The group votes, and this is the group conscience. There's no individual authority. There are no generals or privates in CPA. The leaders are servants. They elect to donate time and effort to the fellowship. All have one thing in common. They're striving not only to get well, but also to stay that way. That's how it was set up; that's the way it works.

## Avoid Domination

Those who elect to serve as leaders do so with no specific time confines. The jobs are rotated frequently. This makes good sense because it offers insight into common problems, allows for the sharing of responsibility, and gives the members some experience. There are always a few who try to dominate. They don't want to be president; they want to be czar. In this case, Tradition 2 must be exercised. The group conscience intervenes. A good group can disintegrate in a hurry when one or two members want to take over. You must keep in mind that ever since God gave Adam and Eve their walking papers, only a few perfect people have strolled the earth. About all you can do is strive for perfection, and some come fairly close. All of us will probably get points for trying.

## Sponsors

Every member should have a good sponsor, and there's no harm in having two. New members often get someone his or her own age as a sponsor, someone with similar problems and a few years of success under the belt. It's also good to find a mature person with good academic knowledge of the Steps and Traditions as well as years of quality success. Run with the winners in your group. Sponsors can be of immense value. One rare problem with sponsors is some become dictatorial; their business, however, is only to offer guidance and support. They must be good listeners. God gave us two ears and only one mouth. We should listen twice as much as we talk.

Sponsors must be able to explain the program and point out the choices, but some get carried away. Tradition 2 points out very succinctly that there's but one authority and that's a Higher Power. Sponsors are not officers in the corporation; there is no hierarchy in CPA. People serve voluntarily with no pay and no prestige. It's a fellowship of equals. There's no discrimination by education, creed, wealth, social status, color, sexuality, or nationality.

## Cliques

Cliques can be as great a threat to group stability as an authoritarian sponsor. A clique can take over a group and the authority with it. The group conscience again must manifest itself and rectify the situation. Cliques, by virtue of numbers, may dominate a group, subtly at first, but overtly later. Tradition 2 should be invoked if the group sees this happening. The work of CPA is too important and the lives involved too valuable to allow any jeopardy of the group's unity. Cliques need to be challenged. The group conscience should make itself felt before damage is inflicted or it's too late. Members who have the perspicacity to see a clique forming need to point it out. They have an obligation to step forward and blow the whistle. It may lead to an embarrassing situation, but it needs to be done.

## Chairman of the Board

Outsiders are constantly amazed at how AA functions. The usual questions are: "Who are the people who run this outfit?" "Who keeps track of the money?" "Who's the chairman of the board?" They're amazed when they're informed that God is the Chairman of the Board. They have a tough time accepting that such an organization can function—yet it does and it does it beautifully. The Philosophy and Principles of AA have not only survived, but they have spread into all fields of addiction and behavioral problems—and yes, also into the management of chronic pain.

## No Hierarchy

Tradition 2 emanates wisdom. When new groups form, they have founders. It's difficult for founders to let go. They need to let God, in the form of group conscience, take over. Tradition 2 is there for a reason. God or a Higher Power, through the group conscience, runs the show; that's the way it must be. There are no trained leaders and it works just fine. The old adage "If it works, don't fix it" should be kept in mind. A chairperson may be elected for the purpose of arranging meetings, but this may be about as far as those duties go. That person acts as a servant of the group. Another "officer" may be a treasurer, seeing that the hat is passed at each meeting. Someone (usually the treasurer) will buy the coffee, pay accumulated bills (if any), and give reports at meetings. The secretary sends out notices and takes care of the literature. Again, all is volunteered; all are servants of the group. Together the officers may form a committee to give advice, judge no one's conduct, and issue no orders. The power in CPA is the group conscience.

## ▲ Tradition 3

The only requirement of Chronic Pain Anonymous is the desire to get well, to learn to manage the ever-present pain.

## Solo Requirement

People join CPA for one reason. They want to be able to function as normal human beings again; they want to learn to live with their pain. They need to share their knowledge and experience with other PWCPs. They need the support of the group. They need to avoid mind-altering agents as much as possible, and to avoid them forever. They need to meet life on its own terms, with their mental faculties intact, not with half a brain. They seek the strength that flows from God and from the group, not from some chemical. In short, they need to get well.

### No Outside Causes

When a cohesive group is formed there's always a tendency to get involved with other causes, therapies, philosophies, or organizations. If this is allowed to happen, the CPA program becomes diluted. It shouldn't be allowed. PWCPs are especially prone to such pitfalls because they have run from physician to physician, hospital to hospital, always hoping for some magical cure. The health field abounds with claims of magical cures. What members choose to do in private or as individuals is their business, but Tradition 3 spells out that this Anonymous organization exists for one specific purpose—getting the PWCP well. CPA isn't to be used as a forum for special interests. It states very simply that only the Steps and Traditions are to be studied and practiced. If they're followed, there's a promise of subjugating the pain problem and getting on with life. Involving other special creeds and philosophies is wrong—it tears up the group. There are no limitations outside the group, but when CPA meets, the Principles and Philosophy of CPA are to be followed. There's nothing new or startling in this guidance. It's precisely what has worked in the past, and it will work in the future.

### No Distractions

The Third Tradition directs you to fix your eyes

and mind on the program, without distractions. It doesn't say it's the only answer. It doesn't say what must be done on your own. It does suggest that other philosophies, religious creeds, or modes of treatment be left at the front door when the meeting starts. "Keep it simple!" is the cry of all Anonymous groups. Tradition 3 suggests that members do not muddy the waters. Concentrate on the program. For God's sake, it doesn't mean abandoning organized religion, condemning quality medicine, pursuing recognized methods of treatment, etc. It merely states the only requirement for membership is that you desire to get well. When in the group, the Principles and Philosophy of CPA are to be followed, and other philosophies and principles are to be placed in the back ranks.

## Churchgoers

Most people who learn the stated Principles and adhere to its Philosophy become regular churchgoers. They return to the basics and become quite often pillars of their churches and communities. The Twelve Step philosophy spills over into their social lives, too. Others make the program their church. So be it—different strokes for different folks.

## Keep It Simple!

You have to be wary of those who wish to turn meetings into an extension of what they consider to be the best treatment therapy. Tradition 2 must then be exercised. These members must be gently led back to earth and reminded to conform to the stated Principles and particularly to Tradition 3. "Keep it simple!"—no tangents.

## Doing It Their Own Way

Chronic pain is a hellish problem. There is a great need for PWCPs to blow away the smoke and return to the Principles, a simple but profound program of living. Those who insist on "doing it my way" often die confused and embittered, worshiping their own intellectual prowess as God. They keep nothing simple. Doing it their way got them into tons of trouble. For many of them, it's time to listen instead of talk. It's time to take advice instead of give it.

### Only One Requirement

Tradition 3 says that all you have to do is have a desire to want help. You can be Public Enemy No. 1 and join the group. To say you want help is the price of admission. Keep it simple! Beggars, bankers, housewives, thieves, physicians, clergy, and some combinations of these—anyone who has chronic pain and wants to get help can join CPA. Most have tried everything else.

Being condemned to a life of pain is not what your lot in life is! In the early days of AA, the founders developed admission criteria. Eventually they threw them out. They figured, "What the hell, some of the biggest losers turned out to be the biggest winners."

## ▲ Tradition 4

Each group should be autonomous except in matters affecting other groups or Chronic Pain Anonymous as a whole.

### Autonomy

AA claims that every imaginable deviation from its original tenets has been tried. Groups have tried to improve on its Philosophy, installed new ideas, switched from one bright innovation to another, and for obvious reasons, reverted to the basic Principles. Today, as always, every individual CPA group has its autonomy; it operates as it very well pleases, as long as it does not affect other CPA groups. The group decides when and where it will meet, what will be discussed, who spends the small amount of money available, and how it is spent.

## No Chaos

This doesn't mean that members have no direction. Each member adheres to the Principles and Philosophy laid down in the Steps. Group conscience decides if there will be a speaker at the next meeting, whether the meeting will be opened or closed, and what the topic will be. Responsibility is not abandoned. There is order, not chaos. Great pains are taken to see that decorum is practiced, for new members are not likely to be attracted to a rabble-rousing group—joining just might mean life or death for that new member.

## Liberty and Freedom

Individual group exercises allow as much liberty and freedom as possible. They are restricted only by the effect they may have on another CPA group. Each group decides how to open and close its meeting. Some say the Serenity Prayer. Some groups open with it, some groups close with it, and some use no prayer. Some just start their meetings with a moment of silence. There is no set format. Some read a Step, some read a Tradition, some do both, and some do neither. There's obviously great latitude.

## Other Groups

There is one obligation this Tradition addresses clearly: "...except in matters affecting other groups." Tradition 4 implies that you can do what you please in a group, but such liberty carries a price tag. That price tag is the responsibility to not affect other groups. Such a dictum is not carte blanche to do whatever you please.

Tradition 4 may at first seem like an invitation to disaster. The opposite has proven to be the case. AA has been around for many years. Millions have studied its Principles and Philosophy. Many have tried to make improvements. The Steps and Traditions weathered well with little or no change. "Res ipsa loquitor"—the thing speaks for itself.

### No Deviant Conduct

"...other groups or CPA as a whole" is an important issue. Groups seldom include the same people at every meeting. Visitors frequent various meetings. Home groups are important and necessary, but experience and a varied approach are also important. Responsibility dictates that newcomers not be subjected to ideas, thoughts, and conduct deviant to that of mainstream CPA. Newcomers will take impressions, messages, and vibrations to other meetings. CPA as a whole could be affected. Tradition 4 is a responsibility not to be taken lightly. Such self-imposed restrictions and limitations may be much more severe than those handed down in the form of a direct order.

### Guidelines

Someone once said, "If you can tell the difference between good advice and bad advice, you don't need advice." The Fourth Tradition advises every group to do its own thing within the confines of its effects on other groups. It's obviously good advice. AA chooses to think of the Traditions only as guidelines. Few would care to contest the wisdom they contain.

## ▲ Tradition 5

Each group has but one primary purpose—to carry its message to the person with chronic pain who still suffers.

## Spreading the Word

Each CPA group is composed of men and women of diverse backgrounds, diverse in age, education, wealth, creed and color, all bonded by one common problem—chronic pain. They understand how chronic pain has almost destroyed them, taken them to the very gates of hell, made them powerless, and twisted and distorted their lives. They understand all this better than anyone. For this reason, people with chronic pain stick to their subject, and they carry the electrifying message of hope to others with the same problem.

They leave alcoholics to alcoholics, cocaine addicts to cocaine addicts, gamblers to the gamblers, and pill addicts to pill addicts. They know chronic pain and are good at helping others in the same fix. They are doubtless good at many, many other things, but on this subject they're the seasoned experts. They've been bruised, battered, and bewildered by chronic pain. They've paid their dues. They've climbed out of the victim's hole and turned their lives around. They stand ready to help others in the same situation learn to live with their pain.

## Living Examples

Tradition 5 implies that those who carry the CPA message are living exemplary lives. It implies that they're practicing the Steps and Traditions. It implies that they're winners. It implies that they're so filled with love they need to bring the same comfort and tranquility to fellow sufferers. Individually gifted people pool their talent and concentrate their efforts on one objective, helping others in chronic pain. It's a priority purpose.

Newcomers learn to listen at meetings. They are comforted. They soon discover that hope does exist.

They make known their needs. They look at fellow members and marvel at the friendship, love, laughter, sympathy, comradeship, compassion, and serenity. It makes them want what the others have. Long-time members appreciate the good news, too, and it's only natural to want to share the message. They themselves have garnered spiritual and emotional comfort, and they've come to an understanding with their pain; they have a real need to share what they have with other "pain pals." They offer a willing ear, a kind word, and a helping hand. They are uniquely qualified to assist other PWCPs.

**Special People, Special Message**

You don't have to be eloquent nor an intellectual giant to pass on the Twelve Step message. Such talent can sometimes frighten less secure people. Some of the most impressive members say little, but they do much. They walk their talk. They practice what they preach. New members come to them; they don't advertise. In striving for the highest perfection of which they are capable, they set an example. They give of themselves. They exude humility and honesty, two of the most important, if not *the* most important, characteristics of a healthy program. Humility and honesty are the basis for success—the sure mark of the winners. Others see it; others want it. Newcomers seek out these special people. The successful members share their success and their message, and all CPA members grow in the process.

## ▲ Tradition 6

A Chronic Pain Anonymous group shall never endorse, finance, or lend their name to any related facility or outside enterprise, lest problems of money, property, and prestige divert us from our primary purpose.

## Grandiosity

There's a natural tendency to take a good idea and bleed it dry. Early AA members knew they had a good thing. Some wanted to exploit it. They dreamed big dreams. They wanted a hospital chain of their own. They wanted to take all their fellow alcoholics and confine them in a specific place, put them to work on projects where they would stay sober and, of course, make a huge pile of money for the organization that could be funneled into educating the public about the evils of alcohol. They also thought about endorsing politicians with sympathy for their cause. The outside possibilities went on and on. The AA founders wisely gave a thumbs-down to all such endeavors.

## No Endorsements

Endorsements often result in trouble. The early AA members had enough trouble. Money was important; few could argue that point but, unfortunately, it would come to them with strings attached. They needed money, but they didn't need it that badly. If they lent their name to related facilities, it could lead to problems. Turmoil, they didn't need.   Money, property, and prestige—all material assets have a way of dividing the best of friends, much less organizations. The founders took a deep breath and stated the principle in black and white: don't fool around with any enterprise, money, names, property, or prestige. Worry about your addiction; if you don't, you won't be around to worry about anything else. The founders had a way of cutting through the non-essential. Equivocation was not their style.

## Tainted Money?

CPA has to be careful, too. There's a fortune to be made in the drug industry. Quacks and quackery abound. With chronic pain, it's open season. Endorsements are still fraught with complications; money is seldom clean. The advice of Tradition 6 holds true today, and even more so. The Tradition simply implies that CPA, as a group, does not endorse any films, books, literature, or enterprises.

## Attending Other Meetings

Anonymous organizations endorse themselves. They may share members as speakers, liaison members, or in other roles, but they share precisely the same philosophy. Generally speaking, it's sometimes difficult to tell whether a person is attending an Alcoholics Anonymous, CPA, Cocaine Anonymous, or Overeaters Anonymous meeting. It's not difficult to see all Anonymous groups interrelate. All you need to do is substitute your particular addiction in the particular group at hand. Cocaine addicts do better in Cocaine Anonymous, but if no CA meeting is available, they can usually get along fairly well at an AA meeting and they always come away with something. CPA members may enjoy and benefit from other Anonymous groups. They may assimilate valuable information and practical tips from men and women with healthy longevity in AA. The primary spiritual aims of both groups are the same. There are only variations of the problem.

## Strength

The identity of the organization needs to be protected if unity is to be preserved. There's deep mutual strength in all Anonymous groups. The limitless fountain of strength that supplies all CPA groups is the Higher Power. An individual member gets his or her strength from this infinite source; the group draws its strength from this same never-ending supply of spiritual help. This is one bank that never goes broke.

## Look To Yourself

CPA simply says, "Cool it! Don't use the group name for any cause or endorsement." Do, however, use the newfound strength to work the program, and if there's any left over, look around for another poor PWCP who is hurting the way you used to. Be grateful, but don't get too carried away. Protect the CPA name. Don't go in too many directions. Keep your priorities in order.

## ▲ Tradition 7

Every group ought to be fully self-supporting, declining outside contributions.

## Finances

At every meeting the basket is passed, and that's about it as far as fund-raising goes! There are no grand financial schemes and no great worries about who has all the money. Essentially, there's very little money to worry about. There are no dues or fees. Each member tosses in what he or she can afford. There are no big drives or solicitations. Each group takes care of its meager bills.

## Money, An Afterthought

There are occasions when money needs to be raised, but that's rare. A raffle, bake sale, or white elephant sale may be in order, but only on a modest scale to cover the projected expenses. In CPA, money is a necessary evil and an afterthought. Financial support usually comes from the group members— pure and simple.

## Strings

Few contributions are ever made without strings attached. Gifts obligate. Tradition 7 states that outside contributions should be turned down. Strings, no matter how tenuous, exert a pressure the group can do without. Over and over, all the Traditions seem to be pushing that same wise theme—concentrate on the basic purpose of getting well and staying that way. Money, reinventing the wheel, supporting meritorious causes, developing hospitals to treat chronic pain patients "the right way," reuniting medicine and religion, agitating for changes in the legislature, endorsing related enterprises, using the media to tell people "who we are and what we are doing," making films, advertising programs—a case could easily be made for any one of them. Basic principles involving individual wellness must always be the first priority, however. Money, fame, and fortune must assume a remote position. Tradition 7 succinctly states this.

## Criticism

The Twelve Traditions are practical tips which have withstood vigorous criticism for many years without change. There's no substitute for experience. They are designed to keep the waters clear. They address pitfalls. The Anonymous organizations are proliferating, and individual groups are gaining in vigor and strength by leaps and bounds. There's a message here. There's a reason for such groups. The group conscience, which is the Higher Power, must play a major part in the success. That's one endorsement the Traditions have no problem with.

## It Works!

There's something about being a part of a group and keeping up your end. People who contribute some money with no coercion feel good about it. When they are financially flush, they throw in a little more; when times are tough, they contribute less. Many are more generous when left to their own devices. Does it work? Time has proven it does. It's not exactly a loaves and fishes story, but there seems to be enough money to pay for the rent (if any), the coffee, the literature, and enough to kick in to a central office (if any). CPA is sustained by the generosity of its members. Nothing could be simpler than that.

## ▲ Tradition 8

Chronic Pain Anonymous should remain forever nonprofessional—but our service centers may employ special workers.

### Central Office

In almost every American city, large or small, there is an Alcoholics Anonymous central office. They are staffed primarily by volunteers who dispense information such as times and locations of meetings in the community. They listen. They give others the benefit of their experience. They get nothing by way of money and they expect nothing. It's Twelve Step work.

### Disharmony

Spirituality and money make poor companions. Medical professionalism, religious professionalism, and advertising professionalism when mixed with CPA or any other Anonymous organization have a way of dividing the organizations and their members. Compromising may creep in before anyone realizes it. It's something any CPA group can do without. Disputes between professionals and nonprofessionals can erode tranquility in a hurry, and this topic is debated bitterly and often. It's one that can't be addressed easily or even rationally sometimes. It can represent a festering sore that never seems to go away.

## Controversy

Most organizations have to hire some help. Volunteers can get burned out with menial tasks, especially those jobs having little to do with Twelve Step work. Janitorial and other jobs eventually require paid help. Conscientious men and women lose lots of sleep over issues like should an author/member make money from writing about CPA or should a cook/member who prepares food and provides clean-up be paid? What happens when there are no volunteers to answer phones? There are dry spells in every group's history when energy and vitality wither. How about hiring someone for those jobs? Should someone be hired who knows nothing about CPA, who has never experienced chronic pain? (Do you have to have cancer to treat it? Do you have to have committed every sin to understand sin?) A "can of worms" is a mild comment when asked to describe the fine line between professionalism and nonprofessionalism.

## Solution

When an organization becomes larger, more professionals seem to come on board. "Special workers" are required. Someone sooner or later needs to be paid. The pay must be commensurate with the going rate for the service provided. Service is service. It's not right for a CPA member to work for less. Right is right. When individual groups become so numerous that a central office is required, it should be supported by all the groups. Some members will object to any payment, citing the Eighth Tradition. Quite often about all the commotion accomplishes is to drive some very qualified people away from the group.

# ▲ Tradition 9

Our groups, as such, ought never to be organized, but we may create service boards or committees directly responsible to those who serve.

## Decisions

Most organizations have positions of authority either by election or appointment. They have "blue and white collar" workers, officers, commanders, etc. Corporations have their drones and queen bees. CPA doesn't work that way at all. Decisions rest with the group. The group elects or appoints individuals to carry out specific tasks, but they act as trusted servants. They invite speakers, plan meetings, keep minutes, lead meetings, and keep track of the money. At no time is the right to direct or control another member given to an individual.

## Service Arms

Service arms or committees may evolve when the size of individual groups expand and create a need. These service arms or committees may require a staff in order to function. As demand dictates, salaried employees may be needed. In Alcoholics Anonymous, money is funneled from satellite AA groups to sustain essential committees and service arms, and this model has been set up for many years. It seems to function beautifully. CPA doesn't need to reinvent the wheel.

## Strength or Weakness?

When an Anonymous organization is studied by outsiders, it seems doomed to fail. Nothing could be further from the truth. Critics forget the spirituality which permeates the group from top to bottom. People who practice the Principles and Philosophy aren't filled with ambition. They're interested in keeping themselves straight rather than taking care of the world. No one gives them orders. Committees issue no orders. They merely suggest courses of action or general guidelines, and it works. A Higher Power must have a hand in it.

## ▲ Tradition 10

Chronic Pain Anonymous has no opinion on outside issues; Chronic Pain Anonymous ought never be drawn into public controversy.

### Goal

Tradition 6 states that CPA never endorses, finances, or lends its name to outside enterprises because it takes away from the primary goal. Tradition 10 goes further. It embellishes the Sixth. It points out how terribly important and how serious the issue is. In essence it says, "Concentrate on your own business!"

People with chronic pain usually have many concerns and they worry over some heavy-duty causes. Tradition 10 says, "Worry if you must, but for God's sake, don't bring your outside causes to the meeting. Keep the focus on the primary goal. Don't muddy the waters."

### Avoid Controversial Issues

Tradition 10 asks its members to take no stand on political issues, religious issues, or social causes. Such stands invite public controversy. The fellowship is composed of a wide variety of people. Bringing up controversial subjects invites dissension and destroys group harmony. The group meetings function to bring members closer together, share common problems and solutions, commandeer support, and communicate experiences—controversial issues scatter members in different directions. Tradition 10 suggests not bringing such issues to CPA.

### De-Focusers

There are some people who come to meetings willing to discuss almost any issue at any time. They're well-read and articulate. They have a wonderful time spreading their wisdom. About the only thing they will not get into is something that tears them up. They turn every subject away from their pain, their primary problem. They give marvelous advice and have great insight into everyone's problems except their own. They are the great "de-focusers." They make poor CPA members and group conscience should not allow them to detract attention from themselves or others.

### Squabbles

If a group does not have its squabbles, it's not composed of human beings. No group can function without some occasional friction. As long as people come together in groups, there will be some infighting. Groups will take issue with other groups—it happens! People are people, and no one is perfect. With all those imperfect people, it seems reasonable to assume there will always be some minor controversies and hard feelings, and it will make for some interesting exchanges. Outside issues, however, are out of order. Who needs them?

## ▲ Tradition 11

The Chronic Pain Anonymous public relations policy is based on attraction, rather than promotion; we need always maintain personal anonymity at the level of press, radio, TV, and films. We need to guard with special care the anonymity of all Chronic Pain Anonymous members.

## Promotion

It's natural to want the rest of the world to know about something as wonderful as CPA. In this high-powered world of ours, the tendency would be to hire the best advertising firm available, assuming there was money available to do so, and then go at it. Millions are out there suffering from chronic pain and they need help. The merciful thing to do would be to get the word out. Promotion through advertisement would seem logical, if not mandatory. The newspapers, radio, TV, and films would be logical choices. Everyone else does it! How can you help somebody if they don't know you exist?

## Attraction

Tradition 11 says, "No, we do not promote. We attract." The program quietly works through its members. Members get well. Others do the promoting. Family members, friends, fellow employees, and others see the miracle at work and they spread the word. Members do their own thing. They concentrate on getting well. They practice the Principles and live the Philosophy. They get well and others witness their transition. As a result, those with similar problems of chronic pain come to the meetings, attracted by the changes they see in members. Attraction is how it works.

## Significant Others

Every person in chronic pain profoundly affects others. These people are known as "significant others." They may not have physical pain but they begin to suffer, too. They often become bitter, disillusioned, unhappy and mad at God, and they need help. They need to form separate organizations patterned after Al-Anon. Al-Anon serves people whose lives have been or are being affected by the alcoholism of a spouse, parent, child, other relative, or friend. In Al-Anon they find the support and encouragement necessary to retain their own sanity. If the people who surround the PWCP become well, they become a subgroup, quietly attracting others to the CPA program.

## Al-Anon

The Steps and Traditions of Al-Anon are almost identical to those found in Alcoholics, Cocaine, Pills, Narcotics, Gambling, and Overeaters Anonymous groups. Like them, Al-Anon operates by attraction, not promotion. AA chose to do it that way. So far, no one has come along with a better idea.

## Going Public

Personal ambition has no place in AA. It has no place in CPA, either. Self-benefiting is anathema. Anonymity is paramount to the group. Substance addiction is nothing to brag about. Even today, alcoholism remains a stigma. Chronic pain is probably more "socially acceptable." Nonetheless, the Traditions discourage going public. Alerting the media about your success is not good. Tradition 11 suggests that you don't go on TV. Just change your life and try to help the next person with chronic pain. Don't take bows, don't expect a bouquet of roses for success, don't do it on radio, and keep out of the spotlight. Let others do the public relations job. Don't worry about tomorrow, just focus on the here and now and take care of your own problems. The world can get along without your help very nicely.

Help those who ask you for assistance. As with the previous Traditions, Tradition 11 contains a lot of plain common sense.

## ▲ Tradition 12

Anonymity is the spiritual foundation of all our traditions, ever reminding us to place principles before personalities.

### Anonymity

Anonymity needs no elucidation. It means staying in the background instead of leading the parade. It means keeping your business to yourself. It means not tooting your own horn. It means attending CPA with no flourish or public display. It does not mean ducking down alleys, switching cabs on the way to meetings, talking in whispers and, in general, taking on the aura of the Secret Service. Again, the Twelfth Tradition is a suggestion. Do what you please about it.

The Twelfth Tradition specifically states that anonymity is the spiritual foundation of all the Traditions. That's a serious statement. Spirituality is what CPA is about, so most members take this advice to heart. They take precautions to remain anonymous. Again, if it works, don't fix it.

### Discipline

Anonymity requires a subjugation of the will. Willful children do as they please. Adults are fond of the expression "The child is willful!" Willful children want what they want, and they want it right now. Self-gratification will not be put off. Some children never mature. As adults, they still operate on a child's maturity level. Anonymity requires humility; it's the opposite of self-gratification or self-centeredness. The Twelfth Tradition is a reminder that to run a successful program, you must exercise discipline.

## Gaining Ground

It requires remarkable effort for a self-centered individual to suddenly graduate from that status to one of humility and thoughtfulness. Two steps forward and one backward is the rule, not the exception. It's a daily struggle, taking a day at a time, hour by hour; but by following the Principles, change does take place. The beauty is you don't just recover lost ground, but you recover that ground and then some.

Chronic pain starts a person on a downward spiral. A PWCP tends to look back with envy at how he or she operated before the pain hit. Most "normal people" have a strong proclivity to embellish and even exaggerate, but that's human nature. If they played the piano before the chronic pain, as they now remember it, they were on the verge of a spectacular concert career. They look back and say to themselves, "If I could get back to where I was!" Unfortunately, things always seem better than they probably were. They pray, hope, and strive to attain past status. Strangely, if the Principles are followed to the letter, these good things seem to happen. You don't merely achieve former status, you run right by it. People become even better and they accomplish more. They attain heights they never thought possible.

## Being Grateful

This may sound strange to an outsider, but many addicts are tremendously grateful to God for sending them the outrageously heavy cross of addiction. Of course, many are not able to develop the strength to carry that cross; they die from its weight. Through the use of the Principles, however, the winners not only develop the strength necessary to live, but they go far beyond. They find life rich and fulfilling—much more so than before they became addicts. They become better fathers, sons, mothers, daughters, employees, employers, and friends. Material goods become secondary. They are at peace and in love with their Higher Power. Of course they are grateful.

## Be On Guard

"Principles above personalities" in the Twelfth Tradition is a reminder that the Higher Power really runs the show. Success breeds pride. Pride scuttles the program. "The Lord giveth and the Lord taketh away." The Twelfth Tradition is a constant reminder that humble people are the ones who win. When members start congratulating themselves on how well they're doing—look out! When they forget who really runs the show, they're on their way out.

## Principles Above Personalities

Personalities are powerful. People with powerful personalities can be both good and bad. Too often, they're bad. Egocentric men and women tend to sport powerful personalities. The world belongs to them and the people in the world are there to be manipulated. Tradition 12 states that principles should be placed above personalities. The Twelve Steps and Traditions, and all they contain, should be weighed against the force of any personality. The Principles should always be followed when they are in conflict with personality. Personalities may be powerfully attractive, but they should always be subjected to careful scrutiny in light of the Principles. That's the message; that's the yardstick. The gold standard is what emanates from the Principles. The Principles should be studied before making any major judgment. Never be swayed by a big voice, magnetic personality, chic appearance, money, or dazzling intellect. As we all know, people can be fickle and self-serving. Trusting in personalities can lead to serious problems. Look to the Principles. Trust in the Principles! People come and go; the Principles do not.

### Message vs. Messenger

The Twelfth Tradition issues an important warning. People are trustworthy some of the time; God is trustworthy all of the time. The Higher Power flows through the Principles. Don't build your life's foundation on sand. Don't blow your Program because another member isn't good or disappoints you. Look to the Principles. Individuals may turn out to be disappointing. They may not walk their talk. Trust in God and the Principles. Use the Steps and Traditions as your guide. Don't discount the message because of the messenger. The group always transcends the individual. It's all implied in Tradition 12.

### Sacrifice

Most successful ventures require a great deal of sacrifice in personal time and effort. You don't build a successful marriage or run a successful business without sacrifice. You don't become a successful member of Chronic Pain Anonymous without personal sacrifice in time and effort. There seems to be a price tag on everything worthwhile. When a group of CPA "pain pals" gathers, in a sense they're paying that price. They're different people with different personalities, but they have one common goal—getting well and staying well. Following The Twelve Steps and Traditions provides the formula.

# Questions and
# Answers

▲    Admittedly, chronic pain is a subject few care to tackle. We have learned much, but our present knowledge leaves much to be desired. It may be of some value to share facts, figures, and general information about chronic pain. Hopefully, Chronic Pain Anonymous will act as a vehicle to educate people not only on the subject of chronic pain, but also offer a new optimistic approach for its management.

Here are some common questions and answers regarding people with chronic pain and pain management:

1. How many people in the United States suffer from chronic pain? What is the cost?

There are no exact figures. No one really knows, but obviously millions suffer from chronic pain. Some authorities claim 60 million. The costs are phenomenal. Americans spend $65 to $100 billion each year. Seven hundred million workdays each year are lost secondary to chronic pain.

Source: Senate Subcommittee on Health, National Arthritis Advisory Board, Arthritis Foundation, American Cancer Society, American Heart Association, National Center for Statistics; 1978.

2. In chronic pain management centers, how many patients are using narcotic drugs?

More than 50% of the patients admitted are using narcotic analgesic drugs.

Source: Boston Pain Center, Spaulding Rehabilitation Hospital

3. Do many PWCPs end up in substance abuse treatment centers?

A significant portion of all treatment center patients are suffering from chronic pain syndrome. There are no published figures available, to my knowledge. Based on over twenty-four years of personal experience, I would place the estimate around 10%. Most are addicted to prescription drugs. Many replace their prescription drugs with alcohol. Many are addicted to combinations.

4. How badly affected is the spouse of the PWCP?

Seventy percent of the marriages of people in chronic pain end in divorce.

Source: Hendler N., cited by Neff, P.N., *Medical World News*, 17:54-60.

5. What is the suicide ideation rate among chronic pain patients?

20% either contemplate or attempt suicide.

Source: Hendler N., cited by Neff, P.N., *Medical World News*, 17:54-60.

6. How do PWCPs get hooked on drugs? Do physicians over-prescribe?

It is not always the fault of the physician. When people become addicted they tend to see multiple physicians,frequent hospital emergency rooms, and become adept (usually) at requesting narcotics and tranquilizers. Easy prescription writers become targets; unfortunately, some eventually end their medical careers facing state licensure medical boards.

7. It seems reaching a bit too far to compare

alcoholism with chronic pain. Please explain.

The disease of alcoholism is often progressive and fatal; chronic pain is intractable—it is often progressive and can be fatal, so debilitating that life is no longer worth living. Alcoholism is characterized by loss of control; with chronic pain, the same is very often true. Alcoholics are preoccupied by alcohol; people who suffer with chronic pain syndrome are preoccupied with their pain day and night. Alcoholics continue to use alcohol despite adverse consequences; PWCPs continue to search for the "magical cure," depleting all finances, self-respect, family ties, etc.—all adverse consequences. Alcoholism leads to distorted thinking, notably denial; PWCPs spend years deluding themselves and denying the existence of the problem. You may substitute heroin, cocaine, pills, sex, and gambling in place of "alcohol" and arrive at the same conclusion. This is precisely the reason for a Twelve Step program in treating and supporting the person with chronic pain over the long haul.

8. How can I tell if I have "lost control" in chronic pain?

The key word is "trouble." When control is lost, trouble comes. If chronic pain causes disintegration of your life—home, work, or social life—that is trouble. For so many men and women, chronic pain destroys home life and completely erodes normal family functioning. There is no social life and often professional life becomes a thing of the past. Depression rears its head. Negativity becomes a way of life. "Loss of control" becomes readily obvious to all but the one with the problem. Like all addictions, denial is a major obstacle in not seeking help, and the more pride a person has, the less likely he or she is to reach out.

9. Do all substance abuse treatment centers and

chronic pain management units have Chronic Pain Anonymous groups?

They should, for the following reasons:

A. CPA would offer a special, sensible, logical, and inexpensive aftercare program that would enhance their other programs and services. Most good treatment facilities are Twelve Step oriented.

B. The success of a treatment center depends largely on the personal success of its patients. CPA, although no guarantee, would make a huge difference.

C. Most of these facilities have multiple meetings going on day and night. Another Anonymous meeting would fit in admirably, particularly if it afforded aftercare where the PWCP felt comfortable. Chronic pain sufferers feel their problems are different and special, and in a sense they are absolutely right.

D. When you graduate from a treatment center, you usually feel a closeness, a security, and a gratitude for what you have learned and achieved. A CPA group would keep you close to other "pain pals," which would be of mutual benefit.

E. The best public relations for a treatment center is always "word of mouth." Newcomers in active CPA groups might seek other treatment in that facility.

10. How many chronic pain management facilities are there in the United States?

As of March 1991 there were 65 inpatient facilities certified by the Commission of Accreditation of Rehabilitation Facilities. There were 95 outpatient facilities accredited. Most belong to large high-powered, university-affiliated medical centers. The accreditation process is rigorous, expensive, and time-consuming. It's also a badge of excellence.

The American Academy of Pain Management also offers a Pain Program Accreditation. The Academy maintains a listing of facilities that meet its standards and abides by the National Code of Ethics and Patient Bill of Rights. For information on pain programs accredited by the Academy or to find a pain management specialist near you, contact the American Academy of Pain Management, 3600 Sisk Road, Suite 2-D, Modesto, CA 95356, or call (209) 545-0754.

There are thousands of "good to not so good" chronic pain management facilities, which for any number of reasons choose not to go for certification. Each city has several such facilities.

11. How many substance abuse treatment centers are there?

It seems as though every other general hospital or every psychiatric hospital now has a substance abuse unit. Practically all of them use the Twelve Step Philosophy.

12. How would someone get a CPA group started?

Probably the easiest way would be to contact a chronic pain management unit or the closest substance abuse treatment center and express an interest. Probably the great majority of new members would come from the facility. God knows they have been treating chronic pain sufferers by the thousands throughout the years.

You do not need a chronic pain management unit or a substance abuse treatment center. All that is needed is a few people suffering from chronic pain, with a will to make big changes and a willingness to use the principles and philosophy of AA to make those changes. They need a meeting place. It also helps to attend some AA meetings to see how they are run.

13. Should CPA limit the number of members in a group?

Usually the problem takes care of itself. When a group gets too large, it splits. People get tired of traveling long distances and start their own group.

14. What are the differences between chronic pain management units and substance abuse treatment programs?

Chronic pain management units specialize in the treatment of chronic pain. They usually withdraw addicted patients from narcotics and spend three or four weeks teaching them how to deal with their pain. Inpatient and outpatient treatment may be offered. They lean heavily on a multidisciplinary approach that includes physical and occupational therapy, psychological and psychiatric evaluation, biofeedback, nerve blocks, TENS units, osteopathic or chiropractic manipulation, ice and heat, water therapy, and appropriate drugs. Unfortunately, most have little familiarity with the Twelve Step program and its application to chronic pain.

Substance abuse treatment programs are primarily geared to taking people off drugs and exposing them to the use of a Twelve Step program. Most PWCPs simply do not get the message in CD programs because they view their problem as uniquely different. CPA, of course, would be a welcome and natural addition to either program.

15. Explain the "gate" theory and its relation to the treatment of chronic pain. Also how does Chronic Pain Anonymous relate to the "gate" theory.

Two Canadians, Drs. Melzach and Wall, postulated that there exists in the central nervous system a mechanism that is able to shut down pain. The two primary adversaries in the theory are substance "P" and endorphins. As long as more substance "P" flows into the CNS, pain exists; when endorphins predominate, the "gate" is closed and pain is no more. The secret, of course, is to manufacture endorphins and therefore shut down the "gate."

Stress and depression lower endorphin levels. It follows that anything which reduces either stress or depression helps keep the "gate" shut. Chronic Pain Anonymous, through the application of the Principles and Philosophy of AA, reduces stress and depression by leaps and bounds. It offers you a lifetime "fix" that costs virtually nothing but your time and effort. Pain reduction is the end result.

16. Where can I find more information on chronic pain?

The American Academy of Pain Management suggests the following materials:

*Innovations in Pain Management,* Volumes 1-4, Richard S. Weiner, Ph.D., Editor (Paul M. Deutsch Press, 1990–1993)

*Management of Pain,* Volumes 1 and 2, John J. Bonica (Lea & Febiger, 1990)

*The American Journal of Pain Management,* AJPM, Stockton, CA

*Pain: A Journal of the International Association for the Study of Pain,* IASP publication, Seattle, WA

*Textbook of Pain,* Second Edition, Ronald Melzack and Patrick O. Wall (Churchill, Livingston, 1989), London, England

*Myofascial Pain,* Volume 1 (1983), Volume 2 (1992), Janet G. Travell and David Simons (Williams & Wilkins)

# Conclusion

There are millions of chronic pain sufferers out there who don't know where to turn. They all have one thing in common: nothing is working for them. They have tried every imaginable cure but they still have their pain. They form a cadre of desperate people. Drugs are no answer, surgery holds no promise; they have little hope. They need support and the type of support that only another person who has travelled a similar road can offer.

Chronic Pain Anonymous will give that support. Within the framework of that organization is a philosophy that has brought hundreds of thousands of beautiful people from the gates of Hades to a life of serenity and peace. PWCPs fight their fight one day at a time. Most of them end up sharing their tranquility. They become givers, not takers.

People ask me what the difference is between an alcoholic and the rest of the populace. I usually tell them that the difference is that a recovering alcoholic is usually a nicer person. I really believe that would be doubly true of a practicing member of Chronic Pain Anonymous. All it takes is an all-out effort.

# Glossary

---

▲

**Algology:** The science and study of pain phenomena.

**Analgesia:** Absence of pain in response to stimulation that would ordinarily cause pain.

**Arthralgia:** Pain in a joint.

**Causalgia:** Sustained burning pain, allodynia and hyperpathia, following traumatic nerve lesion, often combined with sudomotor dysfunction and later trophic changes.

**Central Pain:** Pain associated with a lesion in the central nervous system.

**Deafferentation Pain:** Pain due to lapse of sensory input in the central nervous system.

**Dysesthesia:** An unpleasant sensation, whether spontaneous or evoked.

**Hyperesthesia:** Increased sensation due to stimulation.

**Hyperalgesia:** A response to stimulation that is normally painful.

**Hyperpathia:** A painful syndrome characterized by increased reaction to a stimulus, especially a repetitive stimulus.

**Hypoalgesia:** Diminished sensitivity to stimulation.

**Neuralgia:** Pain in the distribution of nerve or nerves.

**Neuritis:** Inflammation of a nerve or nerves.

**Nociceptor:** A receptor sensitive to noxious stimulus.

**Noxious Stimulus:** A stimulus that is potentially or actually damaging to body tissue.

**Pain Threshold:** The least experience of pain that a subject can recognize.

**Pain Tolerance Level:** The greatest level of pain that a subject is prepared to tolerate.

**Paresthesia:** An abnormal sensation, whether spontaneous or evoked.

**Radiculopathy:** A disturbance or pathological change in one or more nerve roots.

**Radiculitis:** Inflammation of one or more nerve roots.

**Somatic:** Sensory signals from all tissue of the body, usually excluding viscera ("somatosensory input").

**Trigger Point:** Hypersensitive site in the muscle or connective tissue often associated with myofascial pain syndromes.

Source: *Management of Pain,* Volume 1, 2nd Edition, John J. Bonica (Lea & Febiger, 1990)

▲